"A delightful guide full of inspiration and information for those who want to live a full, vibrant, and meaningful life at any age."

—**don Miguel Ruiz**, Author of *The Four Agreements*

"This magnificent book ignites the true spirit of what it means to live fully. But more than that, it provides the precise formula you need to follow if you do indeed want to live as fully as possible, as healthfully as possible, for as long as possible."

—**Christiane Northrup, MD**, Author of *Women's Bodies, Women's Wisdom*

"I have been fortunate to experience firsthand how his visionary view of the human potential actually translates into reality, and I have incorporated his advice into my own life. If there is one book you don't want to miss, it is this one."

—**Emeran A. Mayer, MD, PhD**, Author of *The Mind-Gut Connection*

"The wisdom here is miles deep yet easily accessible, making it instantly usable. What you'll read here can change your life for the better immediately, and you can't ask for more from a book than that."

—**Neale Donald Walsch**, Author of the *Conversations with God* series

"Ilchi Lee shines a bright light of ancient and post modern wisdom on the impact of how each of us defines our life purpose and the pathways we choose for its fulfillment. His book's genius is not only its . . . principles, but also how he infuses it with his own good heart."

—**Michael Bernard Beckwith**, Author of *Life Visioning*

"It's never too late to improve your health, to give back, to find meaning in life, and to awaken. Ilchi Lee shares with you how to do all of this, especially in your later years."

—**Karen Berg**, spiritual director of the Kabbalah Centre

"I am personally choosing to study with Ilchi Lee to 'Live 120 Years' to fulfill my own life purpose. At 88, I feel as though I am getting newer every day! For all of us who are experiencing the deep inner call to participate fully in the next years of the most radical transformation humanity has ever known, this book is an essential guide."

—**Barbara Marx Hubbard**, Founder of the
Foundation for Conscious Evolution

"I especially benefitted from his guidance for integrating our physical, mental and spiritual health that liberates us to realize exciting, meaningful, and complete lives as we grow older. This book is a must-read for all of us who seek to maximize our personal joy and the fullest realization of our purpose."

—**Reed Tuckson, MD**, Advisory Committee of the National Center for
Complementary and Integrative Health at NIH

"He provides practical strategies, probing questions, and the art of story-telling to inspire readers to challenge themselves not only to age gracefully but to become fully enlightened. This is a must-read!"

—**Jessie Jones, PhD**, Director of the Center for Healthy Neighborhoods,
California State University, Fullerton

"This is a book of heartfelt sincerity that offers sustainable and practical tools that will guide you into your twilight years with grace."

—**Darrell Wolfe, Ac.PhD.DNM**, The Doc of Detox, Author of *Healthy to 100*

I've Decided

TO LIVE

120

YEARS

I've Decided
TO LIVE
120
YEARS

The Ancient Secret to Longevity,
Vitality, and Life Transformation

ILCHI LEE

BEST
LIFE
MEDIA

BEST
LIFE
MEDIA

459 N. Gilbert Rd, C-210
Gilbert, AZ 85234
www.BestLifeMedia.com
480-926-2480

First paperback edition: December 2017
Library of Congress Control Number: 2017955288
ISBN-13: 978-1-935127-99-4

Attribution: Poem on the page 260 © 1974 Nancy C. Wood, reprinted from *Many Winters*, courtesy of the Nancy Wood Literary Trust (www.NancyWood.com).

Cover and interior design by Kiryl Lysenka.

I dedicate this book to my father, who was my teacher and friend and showed me what a life of benevolence and completion really is.

CONTENTS

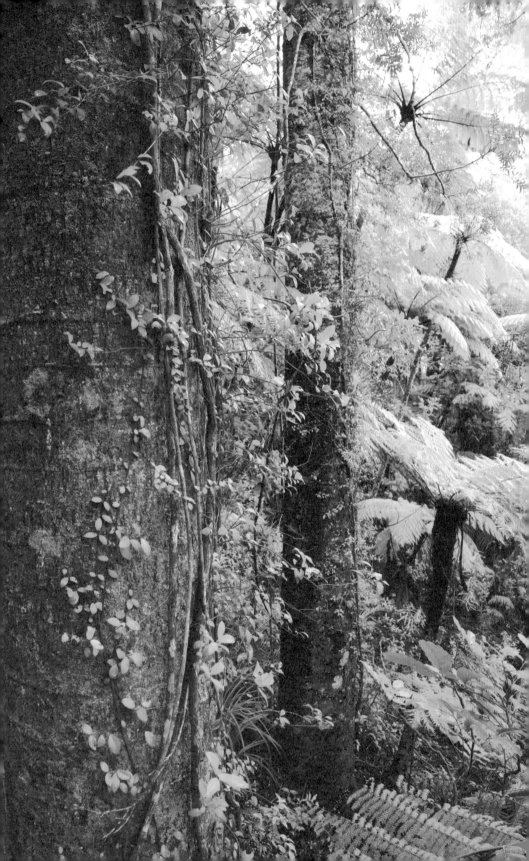

Embracing a New Humanity and a New Earth

C an you imagine yourself at age 120? Perhaps that idea caught your imagination when you read the title of this book, *I've Decided to Live 120 Years*. You may already be accustomed to the idea that you might live to 90 or even 100, but 120 sounds quite absurd. So you may ask yourself, "What secret fountain of youth has this author discovered?"

But let me tell you bluntly: I do not have any magic pill that will guarantee that you or anyone else will live to be 120. I am currently in my late 60s, and I cannot even guarantee that I will live that long. However, I have *decided* to live to age 120.

The key word here is *decided*. I have made a clear, unwavering decision that I will live to 120 years of age. I cannot know when the actual final day of my life will come, but I do know that such a life is a possibility and that I can live my life with the expectation that I will live this long, especially if I take steps to live healthfully and with a deep sense of purpose. Biological research has shown that an individual human's cells hold the potential to function and replicate for 120 years, and maybe even longer if assisted by technologies now on the horizon. It is not at all unrealistic to live one's life with the expectation of living this long.

This book was conceived as I began to look back on my life as I entered my late 60s. I wondered what I wanted to plan to do with my remaining years. In my youth, I thought my life would essentially be over by age 60, since the average lifespan at the time was not very long, and 60 years was viewed as a considerable lifetime. But it's a different story today. People routinely live 20 to 40 years longer than this. Yet, sadly, our cultures still function as though our lives are over by age 60 or 65, and many people over that age are left without a sense of purpose or passion. On top of that, most older people don't know how to maintain their health and vigor, robbing them of the ability to be proactive about their own lives.

Now that we're living longer than ever before, everyone is trying to figure out how to live well in their later years. We're now experiencing a flood of advice for aging success-fully from fitness companies, nutrient suppliers, books, the Internet, TV, and health gurus. But such advice is missing something, it seems to me. It lacks what I call spirit. I believe that the most important task in the second half of life is finding a purpose, one that will give the rest of our years meaning. The spirit that brings each moment vibrantly alive comes from such a purpose. Without it, living even to be 80 might feel boring and pointless.

I wrote this book thinking of readers over 40 who have

started contemplating the latter half of their lives. But it can help anyone, regardless of age, who wants to have a meaningful, fulfilling life. After all, one thing is inescapable: we will all experience old age one day, unless we die tragically young. Planning for a fulfilling old age should be as normal as planning a career path or contributing to a retirement fund. Old age is the future that awaits everyone, and how you live now will have a tremendous effect on your final decades of life.

As I plan my own later years, I rely on the same principles I adopted long ago when I came to believe that it is possible to open a new future for humankind, while also changing individual lives, when our highest selves are realized.

Over the last 37 years, I've made it my mission to help people uncover their true selves and become the highest possible versions of themselves. I founded Body & Brain Yoga and Brain Education for the development of human potential, both of which are based on *Sundo*, a traditional Korean system of mind-body training.

These programs are now being taught worldwide, and my teachings include more than 40 published books and two films. I have met countless people who are interested in improving and extending their lives as I've circled the earth several times a year, going from South Korea to the United States, then to Japan, the United Kingdom, Canada, Germany, China, and now New Zealand.

Now that I am older, I have made the decision to keep going as though I have many years left to live, and to continue working to build a hopeful and sustainable future for all humankind. Two years ago, I started a project in the small city of Kerikeri on the North Island of New Zealand. I am creating a residential school and community there where hundreds of people can experience a self-reliant, earth-friendly lifestyle in a place where humans and nature live in harmony—a beautiful woodland area of 380 acres. This place is called Earth Village.

Through the Earth Village Project, visitors encounter their true selves in a beautiful, natural setting. I wanted to give people what I call "the dream of the Earth Citizen," where people transcend their small selves and begin to embrace others and the world. I want it to be a place that serves as a model of harmony, coexistence, and never-ending peace for the world. I have included pictures of this place throughout this book, hoping that they will inspire you.

I hope you will notice one important thing about this Earth Village vision of mine: it is a vision designed for the future of humankind, not just for people living today. At any age, it is easy to fall into the habit of caring only about that which arises in our day-to-day lives. In our older years especially, it is easy to not care much about the future; we don't feel we have a stake in it since we won't be around to experience it. But by planning to live to be 120, we become stakeholders in the future, and we can live with purpose and vision right up to our last day on earth. For me, by choosing to live to 120 years of age, I can take full responsibility for the plan I have set in motion through the Earth Village Project.

I am writing this book because I believe everyone can live this way, with a sense of purpose and vision for their lives—

their entire lives, not just the first half. Through the years, I have been told many times that my plans were crazy and that I was going to fail. Sometimes I did fail, but more often than not, I have succeeded, and most importantly, I have never given up. As a result, many people's lives have changed for the better, and many people have found their own sense of purpose in life.

As an older person, you may find yourself in a similar predicament—people may tell you that you are crazy to think you can do anything new and important at your age. But I am here to tell you that you can. You can live your life with vision and passion, and you can do something that will make a real difference in this difficult world. It's not too late.

You will learn three important things about yourself and your life through reading this book:

First, the second half of life need not be a time of decline and regression. It can be your golden age—amazingly fulfilling and hopeful. It all depends on what goals you have for your life in your old age. In these pages, I will help you set goals that are truly in alignment with your highest self.

Second, you can take charge of your physical health as you age. You will learn concrete principles and methods for creating your own well-being as you actively manage your aging process. This is not a book on life extension or an anti-aging program, but you will find tips that will help you have a longer and healthier life.

Third, you have the power and potential to affect the future of the entire human species and the earth itself, as well as the lives of individuals around you. You can contribute to birthing a new culture of wisdom unprecedented in human history. It all depends on what values you pursue and what lifestyle you choose for your old age.

I've developed a handful of resources to help you apply what you'll learn in this book, including videos, audio meditations, and illustrated guides. For a deeper experience, an online course is available. You can find them at Live120YearsBook.com.

This book is full of my thoughts and suggestions for designing a complete life after the age of 60. You may have as few as 20 or as many as 60 years following retirement. How would you like to spend that time? Do you have latent goals you have not yet had the chance to achieve? Let's search for an answer together through this book.

I think that the 120-year life is not an impossible dream. It's not a miracle that can be enjoyed only by those with exceptional genes for longevity. It's a tool that people can use to challenge themselves after entering the second half of their lives. The 120-year life is a global project for furthering the progress of the entire human species, not merely a project for our individual longevity.

Through this book, I hope you will think hard about what you can leave behind on the earth. We have a responsibility to make our long lives a blessing for the planet and for the people we love, as well as for ourselves.

From Earth Village in New Zealand,
Ilchi Lee

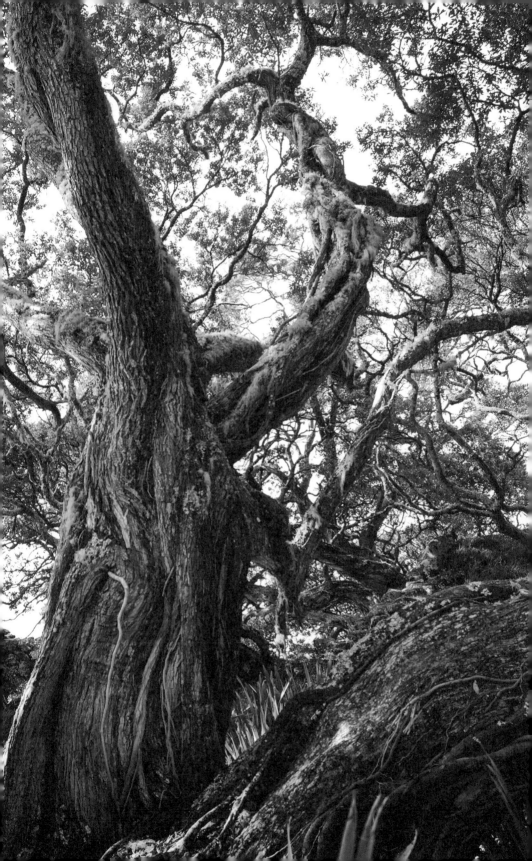

CHAPTER 1

I've Decided to Live 120 Years

I'm 67 years old. And I've decided to live to be 120. Just a few years ago, I thought it would be enough to be active and in good health until I was about 80. My father passed away a few months ago at the age of 94. He was vigorously active through his early 80s. He knew a lot about Eastern thought and feng shui, and after retiring from teaching, he spent his later years counseling townspeople on the sites of their homes and graves, and on life in general. After the age of 85, though, he became much more frail physically and ended up almost never leaving the house. Witnessing my father's old age is probably what led me to think, without even realizing it, that healthy, independent living would be possible until about the age of 80, but that I needed to get ready for the end of my life after that.

In 2008, I wrote a book, *In Full Bloom: A Brain Education Guide for Successful Aging*, with Dr. Jessie Jones, who was co-director of the Center for Successful Aging at California State University, Fullerton. In this book, we introduced the *Jangsaeng* lifestyle, which means living long in health and happiness as you realize your dreams. This book was touted that year by *Foreword Reviews* magazine as one of seven remarkably well-written self-help books. Thankfully, it was loved by many readers as well. Lectures and conferences with Dr. Jones in the United States, South Korea, and Japan gave me an opportunity to meet thousands of seniors who wanted to age successfully. But even then, I had never thought I might be able to live beyond the age of 100.

My Reason for Choosing a 120-year Life

Several developments changed my thinking. For many years, I had come across various stories in the media about the increasing likelihood of reaching age 100 and many interviews with long-lived people around the world. Then, five years ago, I had the opportunity to play golf and talk with 102-year-old Jongjin Lee in South Korea. Not only was he so clear-minded and overflowing with vigor that he could play golf, but his optimism and wit made talking with him a joy. Lee's 66-year-old son, who sat down with us, said that although he sometimes used a golf cart because of his weak knees, his dad could easily walk a four-mile golf course. Jongjin Lee had made up his mind to walk a lot to keep his heart and legs strong, and every morning at six o'clock, he set out on a trail near his home for an hour's walk. When it rained or snowed, he walked with an umbrella.

The experience of meeting and talking directly with someone who was past the age of 100 was an incredible shock to my brain. It was amazing that such vitality and mental strength could pour from the body of a human over 100 years old. After that, I met many other impressive people who were living healthy and vigorous lives even when they were nearly 100. I started to sense that the era of the centenarian had come and that many people are already living it. I started to feel that the amazing increase in the human lifespan was my issue, not simply fascinating statistics or stories on the news.

The first feeling I got from thinking that I might live to be 100 years old was definitely not joyful expectation. It was "Oops!" It was the feeling that I had been diligently running in a half marathon and was close to the finish line when I suddenly realized that the race wasn't a half marathon but a full marathon. I was alarmed by the thought that my body and mind weren't ready to run a full marathon.

I had an important awakening from this contemplation. I realized that I had been thinking passively about my lifespan—in other words, about my time. I had thought only that time had been given to me; I hadn't thought that I could extend my time by my will. I thought that long life was an external thing brought to me by the development of medicine or social and cultural changes; it hadn't really occurred to me that I could direct this process myself.

As a result, I found that my life plan stopped at the age of 80. The time I might have after that was missing from my design for my life. But unless I had a design for life in old age, even if I ended up living to be 90 or 100, I wouldn't feel that I had played an active part. I wouldn't be able to say, "I decided to be who I am and to live for this dream, and I lived to be 90, to be 100, according to the life plan I designed."

After this series of reflections, I made a choice that

would greatly change my thinking. I decided to live 120 years. This is the lifespan generally accepted as biologically possible for human beings. So, I set as my expected lifespan the maximum number of years that current scientific understanding permits, and I then chose to redesign my life from that 120-year perspective.

The fundamental reason I chose to live to be 120, as I revealed in the introduction, was not only a personal desire for a long life. Nor was it a number I could expect based on my family history or my current state of health. My choice stemmed from my desire to be of service to the world and to take responsibility for the great dream that I've set for my life. For this dream, I want to complete the Earth Village Project that I started in New Zealand. This choice brought a lot of changes to my personal life.

First, my thinking about my current age changed significantly. At 67, I'm in the closing stages of an 80-year life, but I've just passed halfway through a 120-year life. I have more than 50 years left! How, then, must I live during that time? What do I want to live for? This shift in my thinking provided me with an opportunity to reflect seriously once again on who I am and what is important in my life, and it further clarified for me what I need to focus on to realize the dreams and values I consider important.

Second, I began to manage my body and mind more actively. If I'm going to live to be 120 years old as a choice instead of relying on just being lucky enough to live a long time, then good health is fundamental. So I work to develop healthier eating and lifestyle habits, and I exercise at every opportunity. For example, thinking that I will need to maintain enough physical power to lift my body, I do 10 handstand push-ups against a wall every day.

Third, my brain has been stimulated, so I work harder now than ever before. The information "120-Year Life" was a new and powerful shock to my brain. Now my brain is passionately searching my existing habits of thought and behavior for anything I need to change, often demanding that I fix things so that I can live a good 120-year life. It has started pumping out new, creative ideas, as if confirming for me that it can perform well for 120 years without a problem. My brain seems to be secreting hormones that increase positivity and vitality, and I feel as though I were 30 years younger.

I feel that my body and mind are now in an optimal state and that I'm living with hope and joy, and more passionately than ever before. I feel great gratitude that, by choosing a 120-year life, I've had an opportunity to design my old age with a long-term perspective and that I now have more time to do meaningful work for other people and the world.

What Do You Think About Living to 120?

Since choosing to live to 120, I've actively spoken about that choice whenever I've had the opportunity, in private or in public. Most people have been fascinated. Sixty-somethings in particular sit back, relaxed, only to lean forward in their seats and listen carefully when I've talked about this.

However, I soon learned that not everyone welcomes my idea. Some have even been antagonistic to my idea of choosing to live to 120. Such people have reacted in one of these three ways:

- Is that really possible? It's still nothing but a dream.

- Oh, my God! For me, that would be hell!

- Just because you made up your mind doesn't mean you're going to live that long, does it? We should just enjoy the years of life given to us before we die.

What about you? What is the first thought or feeling that comes to mind when you hear talk of living to 120? Do you feel expectation or a sense of burden?

The person with the longest documented lifespan was a 122-year-old Frenchwoman, Jeanne Calment, who lived from 1875 to 1997. Quite often we hear of people who claim to have lived even longer, although their births cannot be verified. It is said that most animals existing on earth can live up to six times their growth period. Based on this theory, many scholars believe that the human lifespan, which includes a growth period of 20 years, can be increased to 120 years. Many Eastern traditions of mind-body training suggest that humans can live in good health up to the age of 120 if they take good care of themselves in accordance with natural principles. A research team at Albert Einstein College of Medicine in New York City recently announced that the limit to the human lifespan is 115 years, although many scientists objected to this announcement, arguing that humans can actually live longer than that.

According to 2015 United Nations data, the global population of people over the age of 100 is about 500,000. That's a fourfold increase from 20 years ago, and it is predicted that the number will increase even more rapidly in the future. According to one survey, 72,000 Americans were over the age of 100 in 2014. Not long ago, the global technology company Google started investing massively in a life-extension project. I read one article that said the project's goal is to extend the human lifespan to 500 years.

I'm not sure we can live as long as the goal set up by Google, but I think the time of a 120-year life as the norm could come much faster than we think. The average human life expectancy was no more than 47 years in 1900, but it has continued to increase as nutrition and hygiene have improved and medical technology has developed, and it is now 79 years.

How rapidly is technology developing? Think about our lives 40 years ago. It was unusual then for an individual to own a computer, and we couldn't have imagined the world of today in which everyone carries a smartphone. The development of science and technology, popular awareness of the importance of self-care, and the wider adoption of healthy lifestyles could quickly bring to humanity lives longer than we now imagine. Most South Koreans in their 40s and 50s take it as a given that they will be able to live to the age of 100 if they manage their health well. Insurance products offering coverage up to the age of 110 are now being proactively marketed.

Even if you're not that optimistic about human life extension, it's clear that we will live much longer than our parents' generation. If you're now in your 60s or thereabouts, you could have as few as 20 or as many as 60 years left to live.

Try Multiplying Your Age by 0.7

"Living to be 120? For me that would be hell!" Some who shake their heads at the idea of a 120-year life think, "Old age equals a difficult time of loneliness." Long life brings to mind a picture of sickness, fragility, dependence, and concerns about becoming a burden to someone. Such people may have had a family member or acquaintance who passed away after a bedridden, difficult, painful old age. The old age we encounter through the media is also full of serious problems, further encouraging negative thinking about our later years.

Of course, as we grow older, we cannot avoid the physical and mental changes that accompany the phenomenon of aging. There may be times when things we could once do without difficulty—like lifting heavy objects, leaping up stairs, or quickly learning a new name—no longer feel easy. However, bodies and minds in their 50s and 60s are incomparably more youthful and stronger now than when our parents passed through those ages. Additionally, most of us retire in a much better state of health and finances than previous generations did.

Choosing to live to 120 doesn't mean merely extending our lives for several decades until, immediately before death, we have frail bodies and cloudy minds. It means that we pursue something in our old age, actively choosing how we will live, and we make it a time when we can live in health and happiness, feeling that life is fun and rewarding.

A new method of calculating age was fashionable for a time in Japan, whose people are among the longest lived in the world. According to this method, you multiply your current age by 0.7. Only then, it's claimed, do you get the age you actually feel, physically and mentally, because these days we live much more youthfully than previous generations did. Calculating age this way, a 50-year-old is 35, a 60-year-old is 42, and a 70-year-old is 49. What about a 120-year-old? 84!

Our heads are still influenced by ideas from the time when the average lifespan was 60. Without realizing it, we are programmed to think that our 20s and 30s are the time of our youth, and our 40s and 50s are middle age. Thinking of our 60s and above brings to mind infirm bodies, loss, pain, and dependence.

In many countries, 65 is generally the age of retirement, and from then on a person is commonly classified as a senior. The practice of defining 65 as the beginning of old age is said to have originated in Germany in 1889, when the government paid retirement pensions beginning at the age of 65. We need to remember that the average lifespan at that time wasn't even 50 years. Many gerontologists say that people in their 70s now live similarly to people in their 50s in the 1960s. Rethinking the 120-year life from this perspective will definitely change our preconception that a long old age is a burden.

Life Habits Determine Longevity

As a Tao master, one of the most important things I teach people is that our lives are, fundamentally, not our own. We have received life from nature, and no one knows when that life will leave us. What I chose—living to be 120—is impossible without the blessings of nature. A year from now, even tomorrow, could be my last day on earth.

There is a Korean saying, "Do your best and then await the will of Heaven." It means that, in everything, do your best first and then humbly accept the will of nature as to whether you are successful. The power to end life belongs to nature, but we can extend the time we have through management of our bodies and minds.

Many studies have demonstrated the association between life extension and lifestyle, so those who have chosen unhealthy lives—drinking, smoking, being under too much stress—will have their life expectancies reduced by their choices. Those who have chosen healthy lives—developing good habits, exercising, and thinking positively—will have their life expectancies extended by their choices.

Of the major factors determining longevity, food is definitely important. The food you consume becomes your body. The results of a University of London study of 65,000 people indicated that people who ate seven portions of fruits and vegetables a day had a premature death rate that was 42 percent lower than those who ate less than one portion a day. Those who ate five to six portions a day had a premature death rate that was 36 percent lower.

It is widely known that eating less is one secret to long life. According to one study, people who eat moderately can expect five more years of life. In Japan, many long-lived elderly people stop eating when they feel about 80 percent full. In addition to eating less, another habit seems to be closely associated with long life. Dan Buettner, the author of *The Blue Zones: 9 Lessons for Living Longer from the People Who've Lived the Longest*, interviewed hundreds of people over the age of 100 around the world. He found that most eat their smallest meal in the late afternoon or evening.

The fact that exercise is effective for life extension is universally recognized. According to a study conducted by the US Department of Health and Human Services on subjects age 40 and above, doing 150 minutes of moderate exercise or 75 minutes of high-intensity exercise every week had a life-extension effect of 3.4 years. Doing twice that amount had an extension effect of 4.2 years, and even those who exercised only half the recommended amount lengthened their lives by 1.8 years.

Basic mindset, attitude toward life, and personal relationships are also important for life extension. According to Dr. Becca Levy of the Yale School of Public Health, those who have a positive perspective on aging tend to live about 7.5 years longer than those who have a negative perspective. We usually think that just living carefree and easygoing is effective for longevity, but one study overturned this idea, showing that having a diligent, conscientious, prudent personality extends life two to three years—equivalent to a 20 to 30 percent reduction in premature mortality. According to data from 143 studies in which 300,000 people participated, people who have strong social connections live an average of 7.5 years longer than those who are isolated.

Breaking habits that are bad for the body is essential for life extension. Life is extended six to eight years for a woman who quits smoking at the age of 35. And if she quits at the age of 50, the likelihood that she will die over the next 15 years is cut in half compared to someone who continues smoking. Reducing the time you spend sitting each day to less than three hours has the effect of extending your life expectancy by two years.

Maintaining a healthy lifestyle is directly connected with life extension in so many respects. We can infer that changing major life habits in a healthy direction could extend life by as little as 10 years or as much as several decades. No one can confidently answer "of course" to someone who asks whether living to 120 is possible just because you've made up your mind to do so. However, if our assumptions are based on the brilliant development of medical technology and the results of studies like those I've mentioned, we can say that we are gradually approaching this as a real possibility.

How Long Will You Choose to Live?

To more actively design your old age, I suggest that you choose the age you wish to reach. If you could decide this for yourself, how long would you want to live? Is there some particular age that comes to mind? If so, why that age? Make up your mind to live to a certain age instead of simply wishing to live that long. Express your intention clearly to yourself, not to someone else.

Have you chosen your lifespan? Next, based on the age you have chosen, calculate how much time you have left between now and when you die. Thirty years? Forty years? Fifty? Most people will have quite a long time left. Think seriously about that time. Isn't it at least a third of your whole life, or even nearly half of it?

Now ask yourself these questions: Do I have a goal and a design for the time I have left? What will living to the age I've chosen look like? What do I want to achieve and who will I become during that time? Listen carefully for a voice inside you responding to these questions.

Each and every one of us can choose how we will use the time and the life that have been given to us. This is the greatest power and right that we have. Unfortunately, though, only a tiny fraction of people make good use of this power. Most people have small plans for what they will do tomorrow, what they will do next week, where they will travel during their next vacation, what they will do this holiday season, and so on. Few have plans for five years or ten years from now, much less an overall life plan for where the current of their lives will flow and what goals they will achieve in each stage of their lives— youth, adulthood, middle age, and old age.

Without a big picture for how we will live our lives, and for what, we end up just going with the flow—allowing our circumstances to determine how things work out. French novelist Paul Bourget said this: "We must live as we think, or we shall end up by thinking as we have lived."

After attentively observing and talking with people who, like me, have entered the second half of their lives, I have reached this conclusion: most people lack a concrete picture of their lives in their 70s, 80s, and beyond. This is true for people who are physically, mentally, and socially active, as well as for those who live passive, isolated lives following retirement. Even people who spend their old age in busy activities—traveling, engaging in hobbies, or volunteering—have to-do lists that fill their schedules but rarely have a big picture for what they want to achieve. To design the second half of your life so it is healthy, happy, and overflowing with joy and a sense of fulfillment, you must have a purpose or goal that gives that time meaning.

In fact, for choosing how long you will live, what needs to come first is finding a purpose or goal you want to achieve during the rest of your life. Picking a random number that just pops into your head has little meaning; such a number itself won't motivate you to live to that age. When we have goals that give us meaning, we do our best to achieve those goals, using all the resources we have. When we have a reason for living to a specific age, we work even harder to manage our bodies and minds and to maintain healthy life habits.

At age 73, Susan Gerace of Tempe, Arizona, has a goal of living in good health until the age of 93. She retired after living her whole life as a nurse and nurse practitioner, helping mothers give birth and writing prescriptions for patients. A single mom, she feels great pride and gratitude for the fact that she provided a good education to five children who are living their lives well as mature individuals and good citizens. She said the following about her reason for choosing to live to be 93:

> It was one day last year. I was sitting with my arms around the shoulders of my seven-year-old grandson. He said to me, "Grandma, later, when I grow up and have kids, will you be alive? So you can hug them the way you're hugging me now?" "Sure," I answered. I did a calculation and chose that age.

The thought that Susan wanted to leave behind good memories and life experiences for her children and grandchildren gave her the goal of living in good health at least until the age of 93. My 120 years and Susan's 93 have significance because there are clear reasons and purposes for our choices.

"How long will I choose to live?" Ask yourself this question seriously and listen to your inner voice. You'll find that it is a very powerful question, for it will enable you to realize what you think is important in life. The journey for making the second half the prime of your life begins with this realization.

Today is unlikely to be your last day. But the probability that today will be the first day of the rest of your life is 100 percent. If you reflect on your life so far and plan your future from a long-term perspective, regardless of how long you choose to live, you will clearly be able to have a healthier, more meaningful, more fulfilling life.

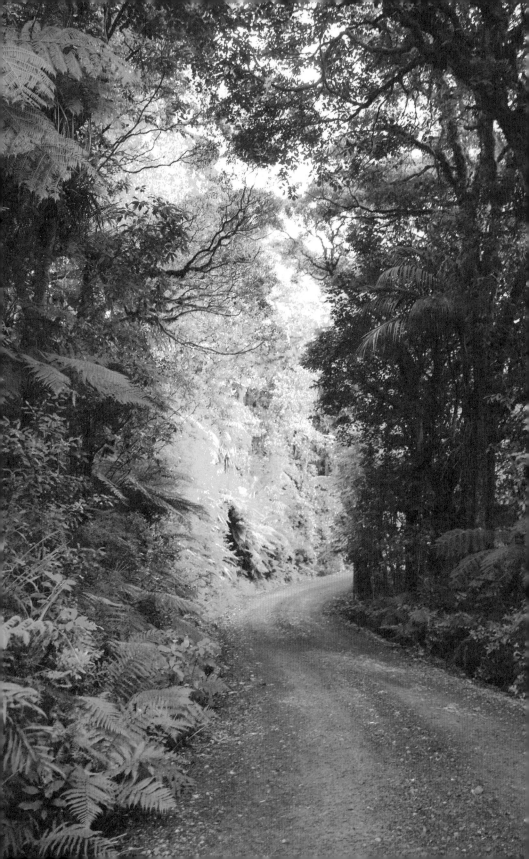

CHAPTER 2

What Is Humanity's True Path?

The phenomenon of the aging society—the result of increased life expectancies and low birth rates—is conspicuous around the globe. The world population is expected to rise about 20 percent by 2050, while the population age 65 and over is projected to surge, approximately doubling the current number. This means that 18 percent of the total population, almost two out of every 10 people, will be seniors.

In the United States, 46 million people—14.5 percent of the total population—were 65 or older in 2014. This is projected to increase to 22 percent by 2050, with the country's 65-plus population reaching approximately 100 million by 2060. The aging society will be especially prominent in developed countries and in Asia. By 2050, the population over age 65 is expected to reach some 36 percent in South Korea, second only to Japan's 40 percent. This means that about four out of 10 people will be elderly, truly an extraordinary development.

Seventy-nine is now the average lifespan in the United States. To see that statistic another way, although some people die before that age, an enormous number live much longer than the average. Look around. We commonly see people living past the age of 80, even past 90, don't we? The problem is that the general perception and attitudes concerning old age remain where they were when the average life expectancy was 60.

When you are 80 years old, what tasks will make up your daily schedule? What will you do on the weekdays and on the weekends? What activities will you take an interest in and focus on? Will you be living with a sense of fulfillment and joy? Or will yours be a passive life, each day a repetition of the day before, as you powerlessly watch time pass? Can you answer these questions?

Very few people have goals or planned activities for their lives after their 70s or 80s beyond simply staying alive. As a result, many people are entering the era of longevity without any mental preparation, and they will face the challenge of 20 to 40 years of inactivity. This is a problem that transcends the level of the individual—it is a national problem, and, beyond that, a global issue. This is a situation without historical precedent: 20 to 40 percent of the total population has 20 to 40 years of idle time on their hands.

The impact of how we spend our time in our old age, therefore, is enormous. If we end up living inactive, nonproductive, dependent lives, it would be a great burden on society. But if we are able to live rewarding and fulfilling lives, and to share valuable wisdom and broad perspectives, we can make productive contributions that pass on the essence of our culture to the next generation. We can find ways to resolve even our own economic problems by giving these activities social value.

By thinking creatively, finding answers, and preparing

solutions together, we will open the possibility of creating a new, mature, harmonious culture that combines the passion and drive of youth and young adulthood with the wisdom and broad-mindedness of old age. Life in old age is an existential problem for many and a reality we will all face, so reflecting on it and searching for answers is imperative.

First 60 Years for Success

I've thought hard about why people perceive old age as a time of little significance, a time when life declines and slowly fizzles out. In the process, I have reflected on all stages of the life cycle, from birth to death. As human beings, there is a path we walk from the time we are born until the time we die. So we cannot help but wonder about the nature of the true path we should walk as humans.

Even at this very moment, right now, we are each walking our own path in life. The details of those paths may differ, but our overall routes are similar. We are born, grow, learn, get jobs, have families, and live until we grow old and die. Let's say that the time up until the age of 60 is the first half of life, and the time after 60 is the second half of life.

The paths we walk and our destinations in the first half of our lives are firmly set. In short, they are about *success*. Every one of us is racing toward the clear goal of success. Success is the paradigm that pervades the first half of life. That's why I've named the first half of life the *period of success*.

People race along the path of life, crashing into each other, flipping this way and that, all immersed in the paradigm of success. Imagine a road of success on which countless multitudes walk, all crowded together. They don't have the time to think about who created that path, nor do they care. They have to make a living—or, to put it bluntly, they have to make a living that allows them to be better off than other people—so they mindlessly race down that road.

The path is now a broad highway because countless people have walked on it throughout the long history of humanity. People don't think twice about why they should walk that path or whether some other path might be available. The road is just there, and since others are walking it, they rush along in the crowd without giving it much thought. They're busy chasing after the people out front so they don't fall behind in the competition.

The paradigm of success begins to be implanted in our brains, consciously or unconsciously, when we are very young. A message is drilled into our heads at school, at work, and even at home: "Life is a battlefield, so you have to fight. And when you fight, you have to win." Losing means failure, so we ceaselessly strive to win. We go back and forth between heaven and hell several times a day, depending on whether we win or lose. When we win, our existential value feels greater, but when we lose, it's like the value of our existence instantly vanishes. Our immersion in competition and success heats up even more as we get jobs, earn money, create families, and raise children.

During this time, we get what we want through hard work

while we contribute to the growth and development of society. We build a career and create a firm social position for ourselves. We dedicate ourselves to producing results through our professions, organizations, and duties. This period of success is a time for accumulating achievements, experience, and know-how.

Despite what we gain from this period of success, it keeps us stuck in the paradigm of competition. As we know all too well, not everyone can win in a competition. When someone wins, somebody else loses. This divides us into a minority of winners and a majority of people who consider themselves losers. In a competitive structure where the fittest survive, my success hurts others, however unintended that may be, and the success of others makes me uncomfortable. That's why there is no true peace within a paradigm of success.

When we enter our 40s and 50s, many of us have questions about the paradigm of success that society has forced on us and that we have internalized. Some have climbed to the top of the ladder in the competition, winning everything they wanted— money, prestige, power—but then think, "Is that all?" They're unhappy even though they are well-off. They somehow feel empty, with no real sense of satisfaction. Even while earning more money than they ever expected to earn and spending long vacations with their families in luxurious overseas villas, many can't shake these feelings of emptiness. Those who seriously ask themselves why naturally end up reflecting on their lives.

For many, the second 60 years of life begin with retirement. Things to which we once assigned meaning and into which we poured our time and energy now suddenly change. Regular income from work, the tasks that once gave our lives a regular rhythm, the intense sense of accomplishment felt through work, the social status that allowed us to supervise other people as we carried out projects, and personal relationships at work that felt just like family with all its fondness and resentments—one day all these things disappear.

People who have sought their sense of worth only outside of themselves, in money or workplace success, experience a great sense of loss at this time. Without the things into which they had poured their passion, life feels pointless and empty unless they can find something to replace them. They feel useless, and their position in the world seems to have vanished.

You were an engineer, a teacher, a marketer, a nurse. What are you now that you no longer do that work? What makes you who you are? When social success is no longer a goal that stimulates and motivates us, what can make our lives feel valuable and meaningful? As you live the rest of your life, what can you do and what goals do you want to have? These are the questions that confront us.

A Paradigm for the Second Half of Life

The first half of life has a clear goal: success. That's why most people feel no need to worry about other things, and there's no time for that, anyway. All they have to do is follow the path ahead of them in a social system made up of family, school, and workplace. Problems, though, come after retirement. The goal of success, into which they put their energy in the first half of their lives, is absent in the second half. There is no obvious paradigm defining the second half of life. The path humanity walks in the first half of life is clear. But that road is there only until retirement. After that, there is no wide road that everyone can follow. So those who find themselves facing the entirely new environment of retirement are at a loss as to how they should live and what they should live for now. Currently, life after retirement is left to each one of us to figure out.

This wasn't much of a problem when the average human lifespan was 60 to 70 years. However, if 20 to 40 percent of the population spend their lives in idleness for 20 to 40 years, without any meaningful goals or activities, it will be a waste for individuals and for society as a whole. I believe that a paradigm representing the second half of life is urgently needed to resolve this issue. We must have something that says, "If you've lived for success in the first half of your life, then live for something else in the second half."

The problem is that the path isn't yet in place. A road for life has been created up through the first half, leaving the remaining second half a pathless wilderness. Only a small minority of people create a clear path for themselves through those empty plains. Most do little with the second half of their lives because they've been shown no obvious way ahead for the time they have left. What must be a paradigm for the second half of life?

I'd like to suggest *completion* as the value we should pursue in the second half of our lives. Completion means everything is realized and to make complete or whole. What do you make complete? Yourself, your life.

I believe that people are born pursuing completion. For example, everyone seeks to connect with others through relationships, which is a way of completing oneself through a sense of belonging. Also, people seek to improve themselves through education and social advancement, which is another form of social completion. They also look for completion through spirituality to feel a sense of unity with the divine or with the Source of the cosmos.

We all ask at some point in our lives, "Who am I?" This question arises as we seek to learn the purpose and meaning of life, and because we want to find the Source of our existence. Humans are the only animals who ask, "Who am I?" And so we pursue completion—which transcends success—at some point in life because we are beings for whom this is inevitable. Our brains are programmed to search for life's true meaning and to pursue wholeness. I think that this is humanity's true nature.

Completion isn't about the visible world or anything external. It is about the world of consciousness, a sense that allows us to feel what is going on inside us. It is a feeling of fulfillment filling our hearts, like pride, satisfaction, oneness, and peace. Completion is finished in the final moment of life when we breathe our last breath. A life of completion is one that allows us in the moment of death to look back on our lives, to feel satisfaction and fulfillment, and to close our eyes in peace and happiness. "I have no more regrets or resentments; I've lived a life full of meaning, and I'm proud of myself." Only you can know whether you feel that your life has been completed. No one else can judge or evaluate that. The degree to which your life has been completed is determined solely by the satisfaction and fulfillment you feel in your own heart.

In your last moments, if you look back over your life and think, "I have regrets in my life. I failed to live the life I really wanted," then you won't be able to feel complete fulfillment in your life.

According to a book written by Australian palliative care nurse Bronnie Ware, *The Top Five Regrets of the Dying*, the most common regret of people facing death is this: "I should've had the courage to live a life that was true to myself, not the life others expected of me." Here are some regrets expressed by the dying: "I shouldn't have worked so much," "I should've had the courage to express my feelings," "I should've stayed in contact with my friends," and "I should've made myself happier."

We want to live the life we really want, we want to be happier, we want to express what we feel, and we want to connect with people instead of living buried by work. The key to living a life of completion is living the life you really want, a life you won't regret when you die. So to live a life of completion, you first have to incessantly ask yourself what kind of life you really want to live.

What is it I really want? I had asked myself this question since I was a child, but I failed to find a satisfactory answer until I was 30. I could have lived without knowing, but I wasn't happy. Outwardly, I was living a very normal life, but inwardly I felt like my life was an empty shell, and I felt that I could no longer endure such a life. It occurred to me that I could no longer ignore the unresolved, most fundamental questions of life and that I had to dig deeply until I got to the very bottom of these issues and found an answer.

When my heart became more earnest about this, I went to Mt. Moak, near Jeonju in South Korea. I began 21 days of ascetic practice without eating or sleeping and focused only on the most fundamental questions, which I asked myself over and over. Who am I and what do I want? After finding the answers to these questions, I was finally able to begin living my true life.

For the last 37 years, I've asked countless people the same question: "What is it you really want?" Answers have differed a great deal. Some people want to start big businesses, and others want to help those who are powerless and underprivileged. Some people just want to live simple, comfortable lives as free of conflict as possible. When I've gone in deeper, though, I've found that there is a common thread running through all those answers.

What people ultimately want isn't money, cool cars, expensive clothing, or lofty titles. It's not material values, like the attainment of wealth and social status. What they want is the feeling that they can live freely and independently, the feeling of loving and being loved, the feeling that their lives are precious and valuable, the feeling that they're contributing to something bigger than themselves. In short, people want, more than anything else, the inner satisfaction that comes from the realization of their highest values.

Finding Your True Self

Lives that are true to ourselves—those are the lives we really want. To live a life true to yourself, though, you must discover what in the world that self is. You have to find your true self so you can say, "This is who I really am." This is the necessary first task for changing direction from a life lived for success to one lived for completion.

What's hopeful is that the second half of life, more than any other time, is optimal for finding and realizing that self. Our lives are so busy while we're passing through the period of success that to survive the competition, we can't afford to take the time to raise our noses from the grindstone. It isn't easy to sit down, relax, and deeply explore the questions of who we are and what we want. We've been busy living day by day as somebody's son or daughter, as someone's mother or father, as someone's partner, or as the title written on our business cards. As our social and family responsibilities decrease in the second half of our lives, though, those labels start to fall away, and we find the opportunity to live simply as ourselves.

We need not grieve that the labels we once used to define ourselves are falling away. We should instead open ourselves to the possibilities that such changes can bring us. We no longer are subject to assessments based on how much money we earn, what titles we have, or what professional fields we work in. No one is yelling at us, telling us what to do, how to do it, or when we have to finish it. Of course, we have responsibilities as elders in our societies and families, but we are unquestionably freer and less tied down than before. We can now live as the people we really want to be, filling our lives with what we want and adjusting our pace for ourselves. What a great blessing!

What is the true self that will lead us to a life of completion? Our real value isn't found in ever-changing external things. External things are always breaking down. Money and fame can be here one minute and gone the next. The body grows old and frail with time, and it ultimately meets its end in death. Within us, we have a self that can dispassionately watch our bodies decline in our last days. My true self is not my name, my body, or my thoughts. It is not my knowledge or experience, and not the things I possess. It is not my successes or my failures. We must leave behind all those external, artificial values and seek the self-existent true self. I call it soul. You can call it by a different name, one that fits your cultural background and belief system. True self, authentic self, essential self—anything is okay.

The soul is not simply a theoretical concept. It is energy and a feeling. The soul is the energy in our hearts. Have you ever suddenly felt the loneliness of your existence or a thirst for the essence of your being? These are messages sent to us when the energy of the soul seeks to awaken. When that energy is activated, we feel it as pure love, empathy, and compassion. The energy of the soul, that feeling, is the essence of your being. We don't know when or how the energy of the soul came to reside within us, but that energy clearly exists in all our hearts. People are only different in that it is still sleeping in some and is activated in others. Although we can't take anything we've obtained in the world with us when we die, we can take this one thing—our souls. Your soul is the essence of your being, the only thing you always have with you, transcending even death. Your soul is the true self you are seeking.

Each of us must find and meet that self. We should be able to shout with joy and pride, "I am me!" We must proclaim that we feel in our hearts a pure self that exists regardless of our negative thoughts, emotions, and experiences, that we have discovered an eternal self that never changes regardless of circumstances. And we should tell our true self that we will do everything we can for the rest of our lives to realize and complete its wishes.

"I am me!" What heartwarming, confident words! Live or die, I am me! That self is the beginning, end, and center of all the values you pursue. Your whole body trembles when you encounter and feel that self. How many hours have we spent in anguish, wandering in search of that self? There is no greater blessing than finding that self. It is the miracle of miracles. It is a greater miracle than healing disease or winning the lottery.

Health and money are here one minute and gone the next, and sooner or later we have to leave them behind when we depart this world. But your true self, your soul, is your eternal partner; it will always be with you. The most meaningful, once-in-a-lifetime event you can experience in this world is finding your true self. It is a marvel that shocks the heavens and shakes the earth.

Your soul cannot be satisfied by money, power, worldly success, or by loving or being loved by a man or woman. Instead of being satisfied by worldly things, it makes us say, "Is that all? So what?" even when everything we want is placed in our hands. Love that self. Love it so much that your heart bursts. Love it to death. Love it madly. Engrave on your heart that your true self is the center of your life by proclaiming, "I am me!"

When I look back over my life, I realize that the driving force behind all my dreams and my vision was my true self. I was able to begin my life for completion because I encountered my true self, which cannot be traded for anything. I am certain that all people have that self, and that all people have a sense that allows them to discover their true selves. It's not that you're bringing your true self from somewhere else; it has always been inside you. All you have to do is uncover it.

To find your true self, you don't need to take a test, and you don't need to compete. And no one else can find it for you. You must not permit some outside authority, someone other than yourself, to determine your existential, eternal value. No school, country, or religion can do this for you. Only you can find and create your value for yourself. Your value is precious not because other people acknowledge it, but because you create and give it meaning yourself. Your life can begin anew with the discovery of your true self.

Expand to the Big Self

If self-discovery is the first process in a life of completion, then the second is growing and realizing the true self you have discovered. Self-realization is living the life your true self really wants.

What does your true self want? Growth and completion. Your true self, the energy of the soul in your heart, wants to grow and be completed. The energy of a soul that has just been discovered is pure, but it is still delicate and weak. The way to develop that energy is to share the energy of love with the people around you. By doing that, you allow the energy of your soul to grow and mature. Then, another realization comes: the knowledge that your true self is not limited to your body, preconceptions, and personality—your small self. Rather, it is a big self connected and one with all things. When you have awakened from the small self at the individual level to the big self at the universal level, your consciousness expands that much more.

There is an attitude that people often have in common once they mature. We want to live lives that contribute to other people and to the world, not lives of pursuing only our own profit. We feel pride and satisfaction when we believe we've contributed even a little to the health, happiness, and peace of other people. We feel that because it's how we are made.

In the second half of a life directed toward completion, we can fully bloom and realize ourselves by expressing the goodness in our hearts. If the first half of our lives was a time for learning, possessing, and accumulating, then the second half is a time for sharing and giving. It is not true that we can help others only if we have a lot of money. People entering the second half of their lives have diverse knowledge, life experience, and skills accumulated over a long time. And they have free time, tolerance, and benevolence as well. Whatever you have to give, you simply have to share it with other people according to your heart's direction, to whatever extent your personal conditions will allow. Your life experiences and wisdom shouldn't remain only your own; they must expand as widely as possible to help others. Share your life and leave something behind for the people and communities who have helped you become who you are today.

We feel the greatest inner satisfaction when we give rather than receive. The influence we can have in the world is determined by what we can give, not what we can get.

Make tight fists and take a deep breath, as deep as you can. Continue inhaling in that state. It will be really hard. Now relax your fists and breathe out. You'll feel more comfortable. The period of success is a time for acquiring and accumulating. If we compare it to our bodies, it's like holding our hands in tight fists and breathing in as much as we can. But no one can continue in that state. We have to relax our hands and breathe out. This is the attitude of life in the period of completion. During our period of completion, we must share and give to others the things we have obtained and received through our period of success. Only if we do that is the cycle of our lives completed.

If, even in your 70s and 80s, you want to live as you did in your period of success, attached only to accumulating external value, then you cannot receive the gifts given to you by the period of completion. There will be no room left in you for inner values such as compassion, freedom, tolerance, composure, harmony, and peace. Your opportunity to experience the true meaning and wisdom hidden in your life will vanish. Don't repeat the life you lived in your period of success when you worried yourself sick about how to get more than other people, about how to look good to other people. If you continue to hold on to things as you did in your period of success and don't practice emptying yourself, then the moment of your death will be terrifying and unhappy. There is no completion for people who end their lives in such a state.

The major difference between success and completion is that competition isn't necessary for pursuing completion. Successful people inevitably compete and fight to acquire more because sharing makes their portion smaller; the material value of their spoils is limited. The inner value of completion, however, is infinite, so your portion doesn't grow smaller when you share what you have.

Achieving your completion doesn't reduce opportunities for others to achieve their completion. You do not become less peaceful by sharing your peace with others. Your peace actually increases and deepens. Success is a race to be the first to cross the finish line, but completion is like a race where there is a winner's cup ready for each runner.

For those of us in our time of completion, the world is no longer a battlefield where we have to fight to survive; it is instead an entirely honest field where we reap what we sow. In this field, we don't need to compete with others but need to actually share our labors and help each other bring in the harvest.

Having been born as human beings, we now face the time to complete the path we walk in life. In the circle of human life that our species has created thus far, the way of success has been the only path available. It has been an incomplete circle, leading us only halfway through our lives. We now need to prepare a path through the remaining half. Our lives will finally be whole when we walk the path of completion. And if this culture of aging well spreads so we all are walking the path of completion, the future of society and the human race will inevitably change for the better.

This new path for completing ourselves and our life is able to change both you and me. I think this is a truly human path, which we, as humans, should walk.

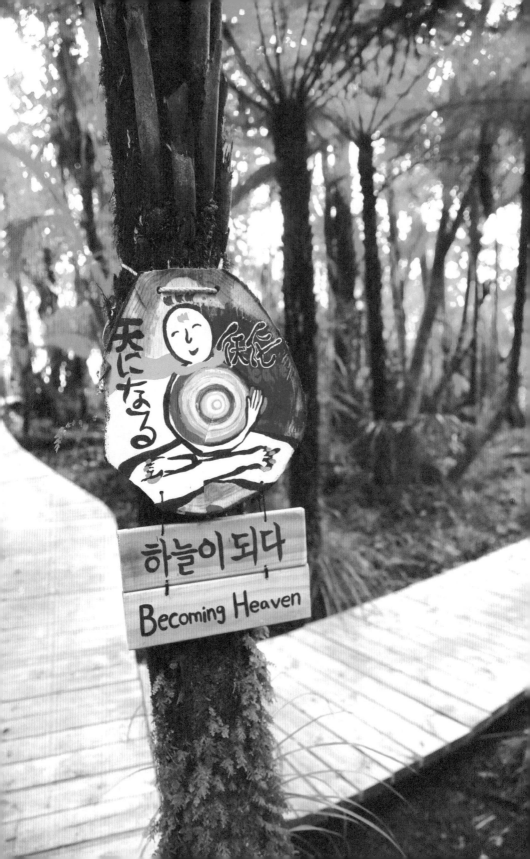

CHAPTER 3

How Do We Achieve Completion?

There is an important milestone we need to ponder on our way toward completion along the path to a new life. That milestone is death. How will I feel about my life in the moment of death? Will I be peaceful, immersed in a sense of fulfillment? Or will I be anxious and remorseful? The feelings we have in that moment can be viewed as a comprehensive summary of our lives. However, the purpose of thinking about death is not to immerse ourselves in negative feelings. Rather, we do so to make our present lives more meaningful and fulfilling. Death sets a standard for us and motivates us, enabling us to live better lives.

The most fundamental worries of old age, the ones that dog us until the final moments of our lives, are about death. Everyone thinks about death every once in a while. As it comes to mind in old age, though, death is a very real, immediate issue, not some abstraction about what will happen in the distant future. When you're young, you can go to the left or to the right, travel paths that are rough or smooth; you have the freedom to choose. When facing your impending death, however, it feels like you've entered a dead-end alley and no longer have any way to turn back. You realize that an unavoidable destiny beyond your power to choose—death—is waiting at the end of the road.

Death on the physical level is experienced by everyone the same way: breathing stops, the heart no longer beats, and brain activity ceases. Not all deaths are identical, though. According to doctors and nurses who have witnessed many people dying in hospice care, how people die is closely related to how they have lived. People who have regrets because they failed to live the lives they wanted generally have a worse time dying. At the moment of death, they may not be able to control the movements of their bodies, they may have more stiffness and pain, and their breathing may become ragged.

Conversely, people who think they've lived the lives they wanted without regret, people who affirm that their lives were good and that they could not have lived them any other way, meet their deaths much more comfortably. They are more likely to close their eyes in peace. Their bodies relax, and satisfied smiles appear on their faces. The kind of death you meet ultimately depends on whether or not you are satisfied as you think back over the path you have taken.

Death for Completing Life

What would it be like if there were no death for humans? If we could continue to live forever without dying, would we be happy? Think about it. If you repeated the kind of days you are living now, day in and day out for thousands of years, how would you feel? It probably wouldn't be all that great. You would have to continue your efforts to find food and shelter, to feed and clothe your body, and to get rest. The daily suffering of having to compete for survival would exhaust you. An endless life of this sort might be so boring and painful that you would want to die as quickly as possible. And the monotony of living forever might also make you disinterested and lazy about pursuing self-development and spirituality.

Death is, in fact, an incredible blessing for our spiritual awakening. Since we know that the time given us doesn't last forever, we try to use that precious time well, without wasting it. We don't know whether some special phenomenon or some other world awaits us after death—death, after all, is an unknown about which no one can say anything for sure—so we try to live our lives well because of that uncertainty. To put it another way, we pursue wholeness and eternity because we are finite beings. There would be no reason to take interest in completion if we were infinite beings, immortal from the very beginning. We feel an instinctual pull toward wholeness and eternity, transcending such limitations, because we are incomplete, finite beings. That's why I feel that death is a great design of the Creator, prepared for the completion of human life.

In Korean culture, there are many words expressing different kinds of death. People who have died after living in ways that only harm others are said to have *dwejida* (similar to croaked). This is the lowest form of death. The word contains a mixture of negative emotions that express this kind of sentiment: That guy lived like an animal. He's better off dead. The second expression is *jukda*, which means an ordinary death and conveys no particular emotions. The third expression is *doragashida*, meaning that the deceased returned to the place she originally came from. This expression is used when mourning the death of parents or elders. Fourth are the expressions *seogeo* and *bungeo*, which refer to the death of someone who lived life on a level that served the national or public good, transcending personal or family interests. The next level is *Chunhwa*, the death of someone who lived a life of completion in Korean Sundo.

I learned from Korean Sundo to view death as the completion of life, not its end. In Sundo, Chunhwa is death on the most beautiful and peaceful level that can be experienced by humans. Translated literally, *chun* means Heaven, and *hwa* means become, so Chunhwa means to become Heaven or heavenly transformation. Heaven here signifies both the Source of life and the heavenly nature that is a part of us—in other words, wholeness. Chunhwa points to the great cycle of actualizing completion within ourselves through the journey of our lives in this world and then the return to the Source of life.

When I describe the concept of Chunhwa, I often use as an illustration the story of the caterpillar's transformation. A caterpillar grows as it spends its days eating leaves and doing little else. It does this until, at a certain time, it stops eating and starts drawing silk out of its body to make a cocoon. After a long period of patience and transformation in the cocoon, the caterpillar one day spreads its dazzling wings and soars through the sky as a beautiful butterfly. No matter how much you stare at a caterpillar crawling along a branch, it's hard to imagine that it could change into a winged butterfly. But hidden inside that caterpillar all along were elements allowing it to become a butterfly. This is the mystery of life, the principle of nature, not something that can be manufactured artificially. A caterpillar creating a cocoon and preparing for the next stage of its life transforms into a butterfly in accordance with the principles of nature.

Just as all caterpillars have genes allowing them to become butterflies, in Sundo, humans are believed to have a seed within them that allows them to reach completion. This seed of wholeness is the soul. The most fundamental reason humans can achieve completion is that we are beings with souls as well as bodies. Physical life ultimately ends with death, no matter how much effort is put into preserving it. That's why there is no completion for the body. It is only through our souls that humans can transcend our finite, physical lives and approach infinity and eternity.

If you want to transcend success and pursue the value of completion, if you want true peace of mind in the moment of your death, then ask yourself this question: shall I live a life centered on the body or a life centered on the soul? Of course, we have to take care of and satisfy the needs of our bodies as well as the needs of our souls—that's our destiny—because we are beings with bodies. The key, though, is knowing what your center is, what you will follow as the driving force guiding your life.

An Energy System for the Soul's Completion

In Sundo, it is believed that growth and completion of the soul are the life goals humans should ultimately pursue, and that our bodies contain a perfect system for achieving these goals. The core of this system is *ki* energy, also called *chi* or *prana*. Ki is the life energy that makes up all things. The ki energy system of the human body is the greatest human technology. It's an amazing microcosm of the universe embedded in the body for humanity's sake.

In Sundo, the center where ki energy is concentrated is called the *dahnjon* (field of energy). This concept is similar to that of the chakra spoken of in India's yogic traditions. Our bodies generally have three dahnjon points: the lower dahnjon in the lower belly, the middle dahnjon in the middle of the chest, and the upper dahnjon in the brain. These three energy centers have their own names and unique energies. The energy of the lower dahnjon is called *jung* energy and controls physical power. The energy of the middle dahnjon is called *ki* energy and controls heart power. The energy of the upper dahnjon is called *shin* energy and controls mental power. The qualities of these three kinds of energy are not set in stone; they change ceaselessly according to our thoughts, feelings, consciousness, and surroundings, and they can always be upgraded by our efforts. The main point of Sundo practice is to strengthen each energy center and raise the level of its energy.

There are Korean expressions that describe a state in which these three kinds of dahnjon energy are developed to an ideal level. *Jungchoong* indicates that the fuller the lower dahnjon is with jung energy, the better; *Kijang* indicates that the more mature and embracing the ki energy is in the middle dahnjon, the better; and *Shinmyung* indicates that the brighter the energy of the upper dahnjon, the better.

Experiencing ki energy with your own senses is essential if you'd like to understand the energy system of the human body thoroughly. This will also greatly help you grasp the process of energy development. You can watch a video teaching you an energy sensitizing exercise at Live120YearsBook.com.

Jungchoong, Kijang, Shinmyung—these three stages of energy development in the human body are important because they are concrete steps for completion of the soul and for Chunhwa. Completion in Sundo is a specific process of development and transformation of the energy in the human body. Once the lower dahnjon is filled with vital energy, it causes the energy of the soul in the middle dahnjon to mature and expand. The mature heart energy of the middle dahnjon rises to the head, awakening and illuminating the divine energy of the brain.

In Sundo, the final stage of this energy development—the energy of the soul meeting the energy of divinity—is called divine-human unity. This means that the soul in the heart, which can be called human energy, and the divinity in the brain, which can be called divine energy, meet and become one. The energies of the soul and divine nature meet in the upper dahnjon of the brain to become one, just as the sperm and egg meet in a mother's womb to become a fetus. The energy

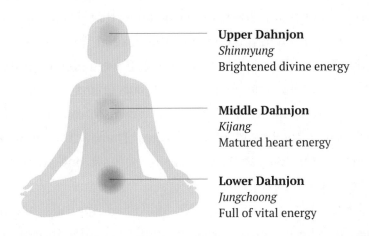

Upper Dahnjon
Shinmyung
Brightened divine energy

Middle Dahnjon
Kijang
Matured heart energy

Lower Dahnjon
Jungchoong
Full of vital energy

THREE TREASURES OF THE BODY, THE DAHNJON SYSTEM

of the soul and divinity that have united in the upper dahnjon experience a spiritual birth in the moment of death the way a fetus experiences physical birth after growing in the womb for nine months. The completed soul leaves the body to join with the great life energy of the cosmos; this is the energy phenomenon of Chunhwa.

What's important at this time is whether the energy of our completed soul leaves through some exit in our bodies. In Sundo, this is called Great Heaven's Gate—the gate for communion with heaven. In traditional Korean culture, people were not allowed to haphazardly touch the crown of another person's head or to pass by the head of someone lying down. As the highest part of the human body and the part that is in touch with heaven, the crown of the head is seen as the sacred portal through which a person received the energy of Heaven. There are not that many people who know that the completed soul leaves through the crown of the head at the moment of death. This is the secret of Chunhwa. If we understand this and develop the energy system of our brains and bodies in our daily lives, we can open the crowns of our heads to connect with the energy of the cosmos. Then, at the moment of our deaths, our souls can easily become one with the energy of the Source.

Divine-human unity is the individual spiritual nature inside of us becoming one with the total spiritual nature of the universe. When the individual feels connected with the whole and experiences divine nature, we call this divine-human unity. This can be experienced through deep meditation, and it can be experienced through ordinary moments in our daily lives. The moments when we feel we are infinite life energy that transcends life and death, when we feel deep gratitude as we follow the principles of that life energy, when we feel the satisfaction and compassion of our souls by transcending our interests to share pure, unconditional love, when we feel that we are a part of nature and experience oneness with nature—all these moments are times when our souls encounter divinity, instants when we take a step closer to completion.

How can we pass through the stages of Jungchoong, Kijang, and Shinmyung and grow and complete the energy of our souls? A road map presented by Sundo points to using three kinds of study: the Study of Principles, the Study of Practice, and the Study of Living. My book *Living Tao:*

Timeless Principles for Everyday Enlightenment covers this in detail. Here is a brief explanation.

The Study of Principles is about opening the eyes of wisdom inside us. When our spiritual eyes open, we are able to see the hidden principles of life and nature. Then enlightenment happens automatically. Such enlightenment should not remain only in our minds as a one-time realization. This awakening to the truth must descend into the body. It is the Study of Practice that makes this possible.

Our bodies are the tools for our Study of Practice, not mere lumps of flesh holding nothing but desires. They are precious vessels containing our souls. Without bodies, we would have no way to encounter and cultivate our souls. You have probably experienced that whenever your mind is a tangle of thoughts, you feel refreshed and lighter after moving your body by walking or doing some other exercise. Training the body is the best way to cultivate the mind. By training your body, you can cleanse and upgrade your physical and mental energy. In short, the Study of Practice is training for cultivating the energy of your body and mind in order to cultivate the soul.

The Study of Living speaks of developing the soul's energy through action in daily life. It's sharing and using the energy of your soul through your work or in your relationships with other people. If the Study of Principles is like planting the seed of enlightenment, then the Study of Practice is like that seed growing into full bloom, and the Study of Living is like those flowers bearing fruit. In other words, true enlightenment is not achieved by just sitting for a long time practicing meditation;

it must be actualized through daily life. When you live a life of practicing, teaching, and sharing what you have realized, then the energy of your soul matures and the energy of your divine nature shines more brightly.

When the Study of Principles, Study of Practice, and Study of Living go round and round like interlocking cogwheels, they act as a powerful vehicle moving you forward to a life of completion. Through these three types of study, the body overflows with vitality, the heart is filled with love, and the brain overflows with wisdom and creativity. Then, you grow as a whole person with boldness and courage, not readily shaken by the emotional winds and waves of life. You are filled with great love and compassion and seek to help others generously and without calculation. You have warm love for humanity and the world and a solid faith in the goodness of the universe.

Life As a Work of Art

Everyone comes to the earth until, sooner or later, they have to return to Heaven. If they know only earth without knowing Heaven, though, they have nowhere to go but the earth. The body belongs to the earth, the soul to Heaven. So our bodies return to the ground, and our souls go to Heaven—but you cannot return to Heaven unless you know Heaven. For the body, without completion there is only death. So your life view changes according to whether you look forward to the death of the body or to the completion of the soul.

The soul is the only thing we can take with us when we die, so it is also the only thing we can rely on to the very end. Another word we can use for the soul is conscience. Only one person can truly evaluate your conscience: you. It cannot be judged by anyone else or by a worldly standard. You are your conscience and Heaven. Central to Chunhwa is the principle that, in light of your conscience, you must be able to feel satisfied, proud, and at peace about the life you have lived. And that depends on how much you have caused the energy of your soul to grow.

There's a standard for the growth of the soul's energy: your upper, middle, and lower dahnjons (the energies of your brain, heart, and belly) must be aligned and feel unified. In other words, your thoughts (brain), feelings (heart), and actions (gut) shouldn't be separate; they should be one, and you should act with integrity. No matter how much you meditate, no matter what great scriptures you read and recite, unless you act on and practice what you know, the growth of your soul's energy will be limited. And no matter how many good deeds you do, if you do them out of selfishness, the power of your soul will not develop. Your soul's energy is activated and grows when you are in a pure state, when your thoughts, feelings, and actions are one. It has nothing to do with recognition by others. It's enough for your soul to be satisfied with itself.

In preparing for life in old age, it's important to know that you can welcome your later years with the dream of Chunhwa instead of just waiting to grow old and die. Although it points to an ideal death, Chunhwa signifies a lifelong process of seeking the soul's growth and completion. Our lives are a process of becoming Heaven, a process of Chunhwa. I usually say this about Chunhwa: "Chunhwa is me saving myself." It's about you saving yourself, not relying on someone else or any external system. The government can't do it for you. Merely believing in something won't make it happen, and no one else can do it in your place. Reading a lot of books or having a lot of knowledge won't do it, either.

What's important is choosing for yourself. You first have to choose to save yourself instead of relying on something external. It's about making a decision: "I will achieve Chunhwa. I will save myself." And you realize that you lack nothing. You have your soul, which is the seed of wholeness inside you, and you continue to develop it. That wholeness grows and grows until, in the end, you attain the completion of your soul.

To put it simply, I want to call that wholeness a heavenly mind. We all have inside of us a bright, pure, noble mind that resembles Heaven, a mind that can embrace and love everyone and everything. No one knows what happens after we die. Although there are a lot of guesses and promises about the afterlife, no one can guarantee them, and we have no way to verify the results. The one thing we can feel directly and know with certainty is the heavenly, holy mind within us. That mind is the seed of wholeness. Continuing to develop that mind until it finally becomes one with Heaven—until it is one with the life energy of the cosmos—leads to the completion of the soul, to Chunhwa. This isn't blindly believing in something, but rather feeling and experiencing it directly through energy phenomena within yourself.

Living and dying without knowing Chunhwa is incredibly sad and unfortunate. Unless you know Chunhwa, you think of death only on a physical level. How anxious and scared would you be meeting death that way? Ultimately, setting aside everything and dying has got to be terrifying. But if you know that there is a flower that blooms in death, the new birth of Chunhwa, then death is a great hope and a festive occasion, not sadness or despair.

Death is a stage on which our souls can be completed. We must one day take the stage of death, which is already prepared for us. Will you crawl onto that stage, trembling in fear, or will you walk out into the spotlight with boldness and confidence? Those who have achieved the completion of their souls can be stars on death's stage. Boldly taking the stage of death—that is the way of Chunhwa.

When our bodies are really worn out after we've done everything we had to do in this world, we need a beautiful, dignified death. A very dignified death, the greatest death, is Chunhwa. Chunhwa is a gate through which we transcend the boundaries of life and death and enter the eternal world. A Chunhwa death is not fear or sadness. It is joy and glory. Our lives become works of art, not pain, when we know the law of Chunhwa. All the mental anxieties and conflicts that come from being finite become a chance to create art out of our lives as we progress toward the growth and completion of the soul.

Will you make your life painful or turn it into a work of art? It's entirely up to you. Only you can raise your true value and make your life more precious. Those who create every day with the goal of the completion of their souls are true artists of life.

Let's Become Enlightened Elders

In the Korean language, there are words that express the stages of life as a process of the soul's growth. A person in the period of growth is called an *eorini* (child), a person in the period of success is called an *eoreun* (adult), and a person in the period of completion is called an *eoreushin* (elder). The common denominator is the word *eol*. The eol can be called the soul or spirit.

A human's eol must grow if he or she is to mature. Of the Korean words expressing the stages of a human life, the first, eorini (child), means someone whose eol or soul is still small and immature. When your soul is small, you think and act in ways that put your own ego or emotions first, without carefully considering others. That's why young children judge and act in self-oriented ways. What they like, what they want to have, what they want to eat—all come first.

A child grows and gradually matures into an adult. Eoreun (adult) means someone whose soul has grown. Adults are people whose souls have matured, allowing them to take responsibility for their own affairs and to embrace those around them. The more your soul has grown when you pass through the period of success in your life, the more likely you are to be successful. When we look around, though, we find many people who don't act their age, who don't act like adults even though they are older. Like children, they make judgments oriented on them-selves and act without considering the people around them. This is because their souls have not yet matured.

An adult who has entered old age is called an eoreushin (elder). Eoreushin means someone whose spirit (eol) is like a god (shin), someone who has brilliant, godlike wisdom. If chil-dren in their period of growth are in the Jungchoong phase when they build up their physical power, then adults in their period of success are in the Kijang phase when they know how to use their heart power, the energy of the soul, in an expansive way. Elders in the final stage, the period of comple-tion, are at the Shinmyung stage, when they have the energy of wisdom capable of wide-ranging insight into the princi-ples of nature and life. To put it another way, eoreushin are enlightened elders whose divine energy in their upper dahnjon now shines brightly.

The terms seniors and old people indicate people who have grown old, expressing only their appearance as seen on the outside. Eoreushin, on the other hand, describes a senior on the inside, someone with wisdom and a bright spirit. In tra-ditional Korean culture, a person's life cycle is judged by their eol, their soul and spirit, rather than their body, and getting older is considered a process of completion for developing and illuminating the soul and the spirit.

Eoreushin, this word that describes those who have devel-oped their souls to have godlike luminosity, teaches us the path that humans ultimately should follow. Becoming an eoreushin— someone who has insight into the hidden principles of nature, who shares virtue and wisdom for life, and who is respected by those around him or her—is the ideal picture of old age, one that allows us to age most happily and beautifully.

Becoming an enlightened elder does not happen automatically simply because you have aged physically. You have to mature internally and have broad tolerance, great love, and bright wisdom. In short, you should give off a numinous energy. Awakening to the principles of nature and life, engaging in practices to develop your energy, and creating true happiness and joy through a life of sharing. This is the way to become an enlightened elder.

I would like to introduce "Arirang," a song about a life lived awakening to one's true self and pursuing completion. "Arirang" is a folk song that has been widely loved by the Korean people over many generations, so much so that this ballad was registered as a UNESCO Intangible Cultural Heritage of Humanity. Here is the original meaning of "Arirang":

Arirang Arirang Arariyo.
You're crossing Arirang hills.
You abandoned me, my love,
but you'll go lame before you make it 10 miles.

Superficially, this song sounds like it's about resentment for a departing lover. However, I interpret it as an earnest desire for completion.

In the word arirang, *a* means the true self, *ri* means enlightenment, and *rang* means joy. So arirang means the joy of awakening to the true self. "You're crossing Arirang hills" means that life is a path into the hills, a path that has many ups and downs for awakening to the true self. "You abandoned me, my love"—these words represent those who go without awakening to their true selves. In the phrase, "you'll be lame before you make it 10 miles," the number 10 represents completion. It's like the Christian cross and the Buddhist swastika (卍)—both of which contain the Chinese character (十) for 10—signifying completion. Being unable to go 10 miles means failing to achieve completion.

The song continues:

O, the joy of awakening to the true self,
Our lives are a path into the hills for
  awakening to the true self.
Those who go without awakening to the true self will go
  lame without achieving completion.

As in the words of "Arirang," let us gladly accept the ups and downs of our paths in life, which help us to awaken to our true selves. Let each of us gladly walk that road, being grateful for every lesson that awaits us on life's rugged way. Then we will begin to see the beauty and loveliness of our life path and of the people we meet along the way on our journey toward our true self and completion.

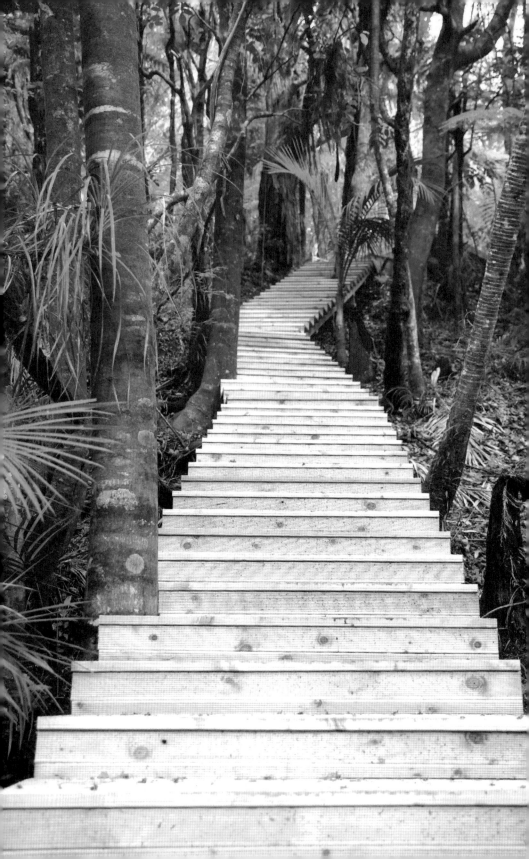

CHAPTER 4

Reflect on the First Half of Your Life, Design the Second

To live the second half of your life for completion—a life that gives you true inner satisfaction and soul fulfillment—there is a process that you must go through. You need to take time to reflect on the first half of your life and to design the second half.

You must fully realize that now is a crucial turning point in your life. This cannot be stressed enough. Will you live the second half of your life merely as compensation for or as an extension of your period of success? Or will you create and develop your life anew from the perspective of completion? That depends on your choices at this turning point.

Many people start to look back on their past when they enter the second half of life. In particular, they become immersed in memories as they recall both good and hard times. But such passive retrospection isn't enough. You must take time to do an interim accounting of your life, reflecting actively and intentionally on your past, with an intention to design your period of completion with a new mindset and new goals.

Renewal doesn't come automatically, and life doesn't change just because you're a year older. You can understand this even if you're only 30 years old. The years pass and the seasons change in accordance with the cycles of nature, but it is you who gives meaning to those changes and you who chooses renewal. Unless you reflect on what you've learned through the past year and on how you will apply those lessons to your future life, aging another year won't make you any wiser. In the same way, unless you take time to consciously look back and reflect deeply on the first half of your life, all that remains will be fleeting memories and feelings. Your experiences won't develop into wisdom for living better in the second half of your life.

I once heard a scholar say that 95 percent of people are living today just as they did yesterday, just as they did a month ago, without anything changing. Renewal doesn't just happen. It comes only to those who consciously pursue it. Only those who open their eyes at daybreak can see the dawn. When dawn comes, it remains as dark as night for you unless you open your eyes. Though spring arrives, you cannot sow seed unless you are aware of the season. You cannot harvest grain in the fall unless you have first sown the seed. The era of longevity stretching out before us holds infinite potential for completing our lives as we want. However, it will end as an unfulfilled possibility unless you perceive it and consciously design the second half of your life. The path to a new life will not open for you unless you choose it.

"The Eagle's Renewal" is a story often cited when personal or corporate self-renewal is stressed. It goes like this:

There once was a village of eagles. The eagles of that village would live to be about 40 years old and then die. According to legend, there was a way they could live up to 70 years, but the method was so painful that no eagle in the village ever thought to attempt it.

There was one brave, curious eagle who liked to soar high and to fly to distant places. This eagle was close to 40 years old and his talons had aged, so he had trouble catching prey. The older he grew, the weaker and duller his beak became. His feathers also grew thicker, making his wings heavy, so soaring magnificently in the sky was difficult. One day he thought, "I'm going to die anyway. I might as well attempt that method of living 70 years, even if it's painful." As the legend goes, he exerted himself and flew to the highest mountain in the village, where he built a nest.

First, he pecked at a rock until his beak broke and fell off. Then, slowly, a new beak grew in its place. Using his new beak, he pulled out his talons one by one. When new talons grew in their place, he used them to pull out his wing feathers one by one. After passing through this painful process, which lasted several months, new feathers finally grew. The brave eagle—transformed into something completely new—spread its big, beautiful wings and flew back to the village. Living another 30 years, he taught other eagles in the village how to be reborn as he had been.

This fable isn't based on scientific fact. It tells us, rather, that the real changes we want in our lives don't come without choice, commitment, and effort. I was deeply moved when I first heard this story. The eagle's courage to overcome its limits, transcend its current self, and be reborn awakens in us a thirst for completion.

Of course, we don't need to make ourselves suffer like the eagle in the story to be reborn in the second half of our lives. However, we must have the courage to look calmly back over our lives and gladly sweep away everything that conceals who we truly are. And we have to choose: I've resolved to have this dream and become this person, and I must complete the life I've designed for myself.

Rewriting the Story of Your Life

There are many ways to look back over your life. You could divide your life into 10-year units, for example, and bring to mind what important things occurred in each of those time periods. Or you could think about what happened in each stage of your life that was meaningful to you—for example, when you were in primary school, middle school, high school, and college, when you started working, when you started a family, and when your children got married.

I recommend that you ask yourself the following questions to reflect actively on the first half of your life:

- What things have I achieved in my life?

- When was I most joyful?

- When were things most trying?

- How did I overcome hardship in those trying moments, and what did I learn through them?

- What moments in my life do I regret?

- When did I do things that made me feel proud and that I found rewarding?

- What momentary choices became opportunities that changed my life?

- What values did I try to remain true to throughout my life?

- What helped me remain true to those values?

- What got in the way of my remaining true to those values?

- What life goals have I had so far?

- What motivated me to establish those goals?

- Which of my life goals have I achieved?

- Which goals have I failed to achieve?

- Who has had a great impact on my life so far?

- Who have I considered precious so far?

- With whom do I want to share my gratitude?

- With whom do I have emotional issues that I need to resolve?

- Which of my habits do I want to keep and develop?

- Which of my habits do I want to discard?

- What things have I really wanted to do but failed to do?

- What were the reasons I couldn't do the things I wanted to do?

If possible, write down your thoughts about these questions. Organizing them in writing instead of just thinking about them will help you unravel the tangle of thoughts rolling around in your head.

When you look back, organize your life story so that it motivates and inspires you, enabling you to live a life of completion. You must not let the story of your past burden you with confusion, hurt, and despair. Use your past as a driving force for making today and tomorrow bright and strong. In that sense, you have to edit and reinterpret your life story. I don't mean that you should deny the reality of the hurts and setbacks you experienced as if they never happened. Nor should you insert good things that never happened. I'm not telling you to distort your past, but to look at it from a new perspective.

Excellent historians do not simply report that something happened in the past. Rather, they interpret what happened from their own unique perspective, pointing out previously unknown historical contexts and providing a basis for action by those who live today. Great historians predict future currents and help us design a better future. We need to reflect on and interpret our lives in this same way.

Don't just say, "This thing happened in the past, so I was happy or sad, so I succeeded or failed." Instead, ask, "What meaning does that have for me, and what meaning does it provide for my future life?" If we're going to do that, we have to be able to view our stories dispassionately and objectively. We shouldn't be bound by or attached to stories from the past. And we must not get mired in selfishness or victim consciousness, either. When we do that, we're stuck as the protagonists of unsatisfactory, chaotic stories, or we turn away from reality and remain immersed in stories of past glories and successes.

The people who deeply move and inspire us, who give us courage, have reinterpreted and rewritten the stories of their lives. These are not people who have lived without failure or hopelessness. But standing before their own histories, instead of simply saying, "This happened to me," they said, "I achieved this despite it all," or "I learned this and moved forward based on what I learned." They are people who got themselves back on their feet through those stories. They became the masters of their own destinies.

Let me introduce an example of this. A distinguished Jewish psychologist in Vienna, 37-year-old Viktor Frankl, was dragged during World War II into the Nazis' Auschwitz concentration camp with his wife and parents. When the camp was liberated three years later at the end of the war, his pregnant wife, his parents, and most of his family had been killed by the Nazis.

Frankl struggled with the fear of death and was deprived of everything he had, the people he loved, and his dignity and freedom as a human being. Yet a single question captivated Frankl while he was living in the concentration camp: is there some reason for a human being to continue to live with constant suffering in an environment completely beyond his control?

"Yes," he concluded. Frankl endured the miseries of life in a concentration camp and decided that there was only one difference between those who died and those who survived: meaning. People who found meaning in something great or small, like a loved one or a sense of responsibility, made it to the end. "Those who have a 'why' to live for," he wrote, "can bear almost any 'how'."

"Everything can be taken from a man but one thing," Frankl wrote in his *Man's Search for Meaning*, "the last of the human freedoms—to choose one's attitude in any given set of circumstances, to choose one's own way."

Although he experienced brutal suffering in extreme circumstances, Frankl never despaired of humanity or life itself. He pledged to endure unavoidable suffering, and he proved that our lives can be full of meaning and value in even the most trying circumstances. Based on his experience, he established new psychological techniques that help people find meaning when they are experiencing anxiety, compulsion, and helplessness. The story of the life that Viktor Frankl rewrote still gives hope and courage to many people.

As you've lived your life until now, there have probably been many crucial moments and events that were turning points for you. If you've had proud moments, you've probably also had things you regret. Whatever life you've lived so far, all the stages of your past life have come together to make you who you are now. What's important is to realize that *you* have created your life so far. Those who think that way can also create their present and their future. Some, though, think, "I didn't make my current condition; it was created by my environment and situation. I had no choice at all, and I was merely a victim." Those who think that way can't choose and take responsibility for their own future.

Whatever life you've lived, it has been yours. All the moments of your life have come together to make you who you are now. It is your unique history and no one else's. With this in mind, have sincere gratitude for your own life's story, and for all the times, places, and people who have appeared as characters in it. More than anything else, love and be grateful to yourself for making it through all those moments to arrive where you are now. Humbly accept all the lessons life has taught you, and turn the story of the first half of your life into fertilizer that will allow the second half to blossom beautifully.

We should live as the masters of our destinies at every moment of our lives—choosing, planning, and acting out our lives for ourselves—but this doesn't mean that everything will work out the way we want it to. Often things go differently than we hoped and planned. That's why everyone is bound to have times when they have regrets: "If I had only chosen differently then . . . ." But it doesn't help at all to sit there regretting the past, for we can never turn back the clock. All we have to do is gratefully accept the things that have worked out well and honestly acknowledge and learn from our foolish mistakes. We can't go forward if we are clinging to the past.

We must never be discouraged or hold ourselves in contempt, saying, "My life so far has been totally wrong. There hasn't been anything of value in my life." We can't exert the energy to start over in the second half of our lives if we blame ourselves this way. If we assess our lives negatively, we come to hate ourselves and to completely close ourselves off from others and the world. Calmly write the tale of your life thus far, but draw hope and enthusiasm from it. Let it be the source of new energy for the story of the life that you will create in the future.

Confessions of a 95-year-old

The earlier we start designing the second half of our lives, the better. As early as our teen years, it's desirable for us to understand that life is a process of self-completion and that success is merely one stage—not the only one—in that process. Those who are mature and have a long-term perspective can live with their own philosophy and integrity intact without being swept away by their environment, even in their period of success.

As we enter our 40s, we need to start drawing a picture of how we want to spend our old age. By the time we're in our 50s at the latest, we should definitely have a direction for our old age so that we can prepare for the life we've chosen. Our post-retirement life could differ dramatically, depending on whether or not we have such a design.

There are many seniors who cannot retire from their jobs

at the usual age and need to keep working in order to survive, sometimes taking low-wage jobs to get by. There are also many seniors who choose not to retire at a typical age. In the medical profession, for instance, it is not unusual to work into one's 80s. Such employed seniors might feel that they don't have time to plan their second half of life and to journey toward completion. However, this isn't something that you can only do if you retire and secure plenty of free time, and it's not as if you have to train or meditate all day long.

The core of a life directed toward completion is the attitude you take in your approach to each and every moment. In other words, it's about what attitude you have in dealing with the work you do and the people you meet. Our life—our work and our relationships—is a wonderful time of study for completion and the best source of material for meditation. If we think about it positively from this perspective, we can say that people who work even in their later years are able to live more vital, meaningful lives than those who spend their old age with nothing to do. We just need to maintain an appropriate work-life balance so our lives are not focused excessively on work.

Not even an experienced architect can build a wonderful building without a plan. If you don't design your life, you end up being dominated by your environment, going wherever your situation takes you. You probably think this way: "I killed myself working over the last 30 years, setting up annual, monthly, weekly, and daily goals and plans. I'm sick and tired of even hearing the word plan or design. What kind of designing am I supposed to do after retirement? I just want to live free!"

Do you really want to live free? Then you have to design your life so you can live that way. Think deeply and in detail about what the free life you want looks like and make the necessary preparation for living such a life. Otherwise, instead of living free, you may end up living out your days without any special changes, challenges, or growth, just surrounded by things that are familiar and comfortable, repeating the same life habits.

"I'll have lots of time. Why hurry? Yeah, I'll take my time thinking about it." If you're thinking this way, read the following words. Printed in a South Korean newspaper in 2008, this article was written by a certain 95-year-old, and it has given many people a lot to think about.

I really worked hard when I was young. As a result, I was recognized for my skills and respected. I was able to retire, proudly and confidently, at the age of 65 thanks to that.

I shed such tears of regret 30 years later, though, on my 95th birthday. My first 65 years were proud and honorable, but the 30 years of my life since then have been full of regret and bitterness.

After retiring, I thought, "I have now lived my life. Any years I have left are just a bonus." With that thought in mind, I just waited for a painless death. A pointless, hopeless life, I lived such a life for some 30 years. Thirty years are a long time, one third of my 95 years of life so far. When I retired, if I had thought that

I could live another 30 years, I really would not have lived that way. It was a great mistake then for me to think that I was old, that it was too late for me to start something.

I'm 95 years old now, but I have a clear mind. I may live 10 years, 20 years more. I'm now going to start studying foreign language, which is something I've wanted to do. I have just one reason for this .... It's so that, on my 105th birthday 10 years from now, I won't regret not starting anything new when I was 95.

This was written by Dr. Seokgyu Kang, founder of Korea's Hoseo University. Even at the age of 100, he would stand at the lectern and share the wisdom he had accumulated in his life; he passed away at the age of 103. Long or short, time just flows by unless we live consciously. There is a Korean saying: "Water flows where directed." Where will the water of your life flow? The time has come to create a new stream for your life to follow.

Change Begins in Choice

When you tell them to design their lives after retirement, many people first think of things like putting together a nest egg, making travel plans, finding a senior community where they'll live in their old age, and—further off—setting up a will and establishing guidelines for a funeral. But what's most important before these concrete details is to think deeply about what meaning your post-retirement life has for you and to have the dream of completion. Only if you have an overarching direction can you use your remaining time independently and creatively. More than simply creating a bucket list or a to-do list, this is about choosing a direction for the second half of your life. If that direction is clear, you can find concrete ways to reach your intended destination.

The outside world is overflowing with information about how to live after retirement. TV commercials tell us to spend our money on maintaining our youth, beauty, and vigor. Investors and insurance companies say, "Entrust us with your money and health while you enjoy a sailboat and a romantic beach." "Trust me," politicians advise. "I'll create policies that will keep you safe in your old age." Information comes from the outside, but it also wells up from within. What kind of information are you giving yourself about the life you have left? What messages are you sending yourself about your future?

It is desirable and commendable to take good care of your body so that when you're older, your muscles don't lose their strength, your skin doesn't wrinkle so much, and you maintain healthy hearing and eyesight for as long as possible. You can also make use of modern medicine to spend your old age with greater vigor. For example, my eyesight declined a great deal as I approached 60. Constantly putting on and taking off my glasses was a pain, so I had laser eye surgery. My teeth were weak and my gums hurt, so I also got several implants. But our bodies age with time no matter how well we take care of them, and it is also wise to accept gladly a body that's aging in accordance with the principles of nature.

We have something that never ages, though: our spirit. The great spirit that wells up from within human beings—that free, creative consciousness—never ages no matter how old we get. That spirit encourages us, asking us who we are and allowing us to spend our time meaningfully until the last moment of life. Those who encounter their spirit and live according to its guidance are not slaves to their environment. They are the masters of their destiny. What we need most for a healthy, happy old age isn't a financial expert or a coach to create exercise programs and diets for us. What we need most is to listen to our own inner voices, our souls, and to choose how we really want to live and what sort of people we will be.

Where should you begin? Begin by asking yourself a question. What is the life your soul wants, beyond the answers set by the world? And ask yourself what's in your heart, not your head. Ask again and again what it is that you earnestly want in your heart and what kind of life will bring real joy to your soul. If you close your eyes and go within, following the feelings in your heart, at some moment the answer will come to you. Once you've found it, resolve to do your best to realize the dream you really want, making the most of this new, precious time that has been given to you.

All changes begin with a choice. We may fail many times, sometimes because of the ups and downs of life beyond our control, sometimes because of our laziness, fears, and habits. However, we draw closer to the life we choose, step by step, when we choose and act sincerely, without giving up. *We can make choices.* This is something truly precious. Even seemingly difficult changes begin with choosing to pursue them. Whatever surroundings you find yourself in, you can choose to improve that environment, even if only a little. As we age, we face new changes in our environment, such as weakening bodies, retirement, and separation. Many people accept such changes as restrictions and limitations, and they are dispirited by the thought that they can't do anything about them. But as long as our souls are awakened, we can choose and create change in any environment.

We each captain the ships of our own lives. We can drift through life, or we can make life an epic voyage. One thing decides that: whether or not you know where you are going. You are the only one who can choose that direction. The power to look back on our lives, to reflect, to dream, and to choose to be a certain way—this is a gift given only to humans. That power doesn't disappear just because we grow older. It can actually grow stronger with age because, as we've navigated life's stormy waters, we have lived long enough to know all too well that we alone can pioneer and take responsibility for our own lives. Until the final moment of our voyage, we should go forward, never holding back on this beautiful power.

I made my choice to live to 120 as I walked a woodland path in Earth Village in Kerikeri, New Zealand. It takes about one hour to slowly walk this beautiful forest trail, which I've named The Way of New Life. There is a steep hill about halfway through the trail, which we use as a walking meditation course, and on that hill I installed wooden stairs to prevent damage to the exposed tree roots and to keep people from tripping on the roots.

I insisted on 120 steps, because I hoped that those who climbed them would awaken to their own infinite value as they communed with nature, that they would have the great dream of contributing to a healthier, more beautiful, more peaceful earth, and that they would choose to live to be 120 years old.

The stairway continues without a break until the 60th step, which has a broad wooden deck to the right. This is the halfway point, with the first 60 steps representing the first half of life and the remaining 60 steps representing the second half. The wooden deck in the middle symbolizes the transition period when we move on to our second 60 years. Although there will be differences from person to person, generally the time when we retire from work life can be called a transition period.

I call the first 60 years your congenital destiny and the next 60 years your acquired destiny. Your congenital destiny is the destiny you were born with and the one the world has constantly imposed on you, and your acquired destiny is the destiny you create for yourself by your own choices and effort. Of course, we can shape our destiny with our choices and actions at any age, but in the first 60 years, we are likely to live within society's rules, even when they are counter to our soul's yearning. In the second 60 years, we are about to embark on a new destiny driven by our soul's deepest desires and run by our own rules.

Depending on what choices and designs you make right at this moment for today, your day will definitely change. In the same way, it hardly needs to be restated that your choices impact your lifespan as well as your quality of life in old age. Our ultimate destiny is up to nature, but we are the ones who work out the details. It's important to open our eyes to the free will and power of choice that have been given to us. And we will be able to encounter a new path in life—an amazing acquired destiny—if we continue to change our day-to-day destiny according to a long-term design for life.

Provide Your Own Health, Happiness, and Peace

Everyone should keep this one precept in mind when designing the second half of a life centered on the value of completion: you have to create your own health, happiness, and peace; you cannot rely on someone else to provide them. If you are responsible for your health, happiness, and peace and take an active approach toward enhancing them, a longer lifespan will follow naturally.

Think about it. How could you hope to live to be 100 or 120 years old by relying on your external environment—on other people or systems—for your health, happiness, and peace? Not only is that being greedy, but you'd become a burden to others. It would undoubtedly be troubling to see yourself as a burden, and you might consider it better to close your eyes early instead. My point is that even when you're older, you should be self-sufficient in health, happiness, and peace.

If you look around, though, you'll see that many people tend to rely on externals instead of being self-sufficient for these things. Just looking at health, we see that people go to a pharmacy or hospital when they're just a little sick. You can get medical help when necessary, of course, but neither doctors nor medicines guarantee the fundamentals of our health like muscle strength, lung capacity, sense of balance, reflexes, and immunity. A healthy constitution is not something anyone else can develop for you. You have to develop it through your own strength.

The same thing goes for happiness and peace. Many people rely on externals to provide these. They feel happy when they get something they want or when someone gives them support and praise. But if you rely on external conditions, it's easy for happiness to end and unhappiness to begin as soon as that object or person disappears. It's like living on a tightrope, swayed by an external environment that pushes you back and forth between happiness and unhappiness, moment by moment. We can become the true masters of our health, happiness, and peace when we learn how to create them for ourselves instead of relying on the outside environment, begging for them and hoping that they'll come. Furthermore, once you're centered in health, happiness, and peace, you can share them with others as well.

How are you doing right now? If you were told to score yourself for health, happiness, and peace, how many points out of 100 would you give yourself for each of them? Are you self-sufficient in these things, or do you tend to rely on your external environment for them? Score yourself after thinking about it carefully. This isn't an objective index but rather a way to assess yourself based on your subjective feelings, thoughts, and satisfaction.

- Am I healthy? ___ points
- Do I provide myself with my own health? ___ points
- Am I happy? ___ points
- Do I provide myself with my own happiness? ___ points
- Am I peaceful? ___ points
- Do I provide myself with my own peace? ___ points

There's no need to be disappointed if your scores are low. It's not too late. All you have to do is begin now. You always have hope, because health, happiness, and peace are definitely variable and achievable and because they are energy phenomena arising in our bodies. They are not remote qualities that can be obtained only through great effort.

To provide for your own health, happiness, and peace, you need to train your physical power, heart power, and brain power. Physical power is a cornerstone for happiness and health in old age. Developing physical power is also a shortcut for developing heart power and brain power. If you don't know where or how to begin designing your old age, try starting with physical power. When your body develops strength, your ambition naturally grows along with it, and you find that you have new ideas and new things you want to try. It's a good idea to find a concrete physical goal for the level of physical power you want to reach or an ideal model you can imitate.

Your heart power grows when you have core values that guide your life. You choose words and actions in keeping with your soul and conscience, you try to reveal fully the positive character qualities within you, and you have mature sentiments. Like your physical power, the more you use the power of your heart, the greater it grows. Heart power is a strength that develops through relationships. The tolerance, compassion, understanding, forgiveness, and consideration within us grow when we train them, just as we train to increase our physical power. Close personal relationships such as those with family and friends and the communities to which we belong are excellent training grounds for heart power.

The core of brain power is creativity. Having lots of knowledge does not mean that you have strong brain power. Brain power uses insight and wisdom to create something that contributes to ourselves and to the world. "Necessity is the mother of invention," the saying goes. This expresses very well how creativity, a characteristic of the brain, is manifested. Creativity comes from curiosity, from interest in and love for ourselves and the world. If you carefully examine yourself and what's around you with affection, then ideas on how to fix and improve things are bound to come to mind. Acting on these ideas with will and focus leads to creation.

A life of completion begins with providing for your own health, happiness, and peace by developing physical power, heart power, and brain power. This is consistent with the process for developing the body's energy system to achieve spiritual completion in Korea's Sundo tradition. When the lower dahnjon in the belly is sufficiently developed, it becomes the source of reliable physical power, and the body's vital energy is strengthened. When the middle dahnjon in the heart is developed, heart power grows, and virtues such as love, tolerance, and empathy are expressed. When the upper dahnjon in the head is developed, brain power grows, and insight, understanding, and wisdom develop.

In the following chapters, I will introduce concrete methods to help you design your life beautifully in old age—in a way that is directed toward completion as you provide for your own health, happiness, and peace.

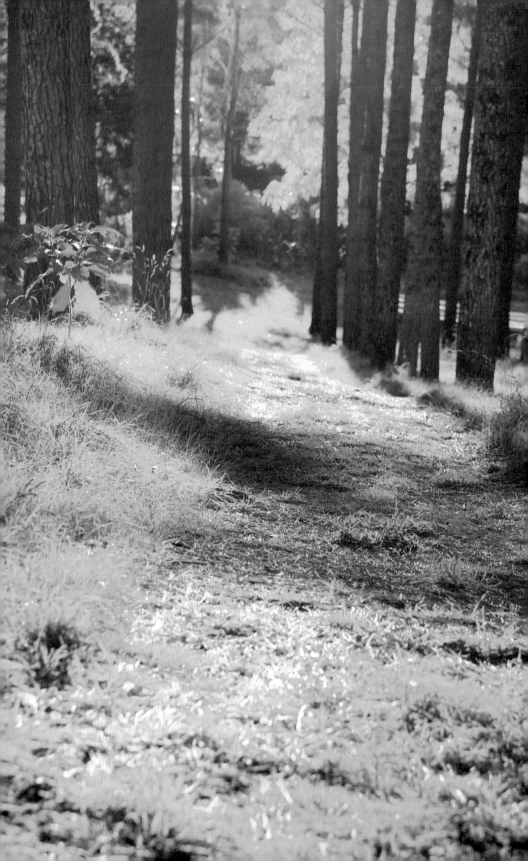

CHAPTER 5

Physical Power Is Life—Just Move

If you asked me what we need to take care of first to provide ourselves with health, happiness, and peace, it would be health. Health is a springboard and shortcut to happiness and peace. "Physical power is life," I say. Physical power is proportional to your life force, so improving your physical condition is the best way to extend your life force. To live to be 120 years old, you need to put effort into improving your physical condition.

The obstacles many people face, however, were driven home for me when I saw statistics on the status of health and healthcare in the United States. Currently, 87 percent of US adults over the age of 65 have at least one chronic illness, while 68 percent have two or more. In comparison, 33 percent of adults over 65 in the United Kingdom and 56 percent in Canada have two or more chronic conditions. Out of 224 countries, the United States ranks 31st in life expectancy in 2015.

To treat their illnesses, Americans rely heavily on medications—more than any other nation in the world. Although the United States holds just 5 percent of the world's population, it consumes 75 percent of the world's prescription drugs. Overall, the United States spends more money on healthcare per capita than any other country ($9,507 per capita GDP in the United States vs. $3,763 per capita on average in Organisation for Economic Co-operation and Development (OECD) countries in 2017). Unfortunately, healthcare costs can be too much for some individuals. According to one Harvard University study, healthcare spending accounts for 62 percent of bankruptcies in the United States. Among those who filed for bankruptcy due to medical expenses, 72 percent even had health insurance.

The way to counteract the current situation, I believe, is to focus on your own self-care and to become more self-sufficient and less dependent on healthcare institutions. By using your own body to heal your body on a daily basis, you can reduce or eliminate your need for medical treatment.

This is possible because, ultimately, diseases share a single root. They always arise from blockage in the flow of energy, preventing an organism from accessing its original, natural healing power. Conditions causing most symptoms recover with time, if you release blockages and restore good blood and energy circulation. Although we can't do anything about some factors, including genetics, others can be controlled. If you grow closer to your body, you can't help but grow distant from hospitals and pharmacies. People who go to hospitals and pharmacies usually keep returning to them every time they feel ill. But we don't need to rely on hospitals or medications every time we hurt a little. We should work to develop our own physical condition, telling ourselves, "When it comes to my body, I am the primary doctor." With will and effort, you can live a long, youthful, healthy life.

Exercise is truly a supplement that has a powerful effect; it's an exceptional method for enhancing life expectancy, health, and energy levels. According to one Canadian study, even people in their 50s who have never exercised regularly before can reduce their biological age by roughly 10 years by walking at a fast pace for about 30 minutes three times a week.

The effects of exercise are innumerable, but it especially helps slow down sarcopenia (muscle loss in old age). Your muscles begin to deteriorate as early as your 30s, but the greatest changes happen in your 40s and 50s. By your 90s, your muscle mass has decreased by almost 50 percent compared to your 20s, and in your 70s your strength has likely decreased 30 percent compared to your 50s. Exercise is the most important way to deal with sarcopenia. Resistance training and strength training are particularly effective.

When I looked at my father as he got older, I often felt sorry for him. He was quite healthy as late as his 80s, but past the age of 90, he slowed down significantly and his speech declined. When I touched his body with my hand, attempting to teach him some exercise, he would flatly refuse. All I could do for him was recommend good food, massage his arms and legs, and apply cream to the age spots on his face. I thought as I looked at Dad that I should have taught him some exercises to manage his health, at least when he was in his 80s. In his 90s, his physical power and endurance were so weak that it wouldn't have been easy to develop a habit of exercising.

The younger you are when you develop the habit of taking care of your physical strength, the better. But it's never too late to start. "The old are weak" is merely a socially accepted myth. Everyone becomes weaker if they don't develop and use their strength. Many older people suffer from stiffness of joints, muscle, and connective tissue, along with loss of balance. The best way to improve these symptoms is to move your body and exercise. It's up to you whether you will just stand by, lamenting the decline of your body, or move actively and build your physical strength. You will grow stronger if you develop and use your strength, even when you're older. Let me give you an example.

The protagonist of the story is 105-year-old French cyclist Robert Marchand. Born in northern France in 1911, he made a living in many professions, switching from fireman to truck driver, lumberjack, and farmer. He had done some cycling when he was young, but he was 67 years old when he started again in earnest. In January 2017, at the age of 105, he set a new world record, completing a 22-kilometer course in one hour. His maximum oxygen uptake (VO_2 max), heart rate, and heart and lung health were measured over two years, and it was discovered that his aerobic capacity was that of a 50-year-old, some 55 years younger than his actual age. Even more amazing was the fact that his VO_2 max increased 13 percent.

My eyes popped when I read about him. Unless you're a professional cyclist, it wouldn't be easy to cover 22 kilometers in one hour, even if you were young. It was shocking that he was able to maintain such health and vitality to the age of 105.

I printed a picture of him cycling and attached it to the front of my desk. It's there to give me hope and stimulation every time I see it. I hope that I can break the fixed idea that the body grows weak with age and develop my own physical condition.

We occasionally hear about people who are said to be the oldest in the world. What amazes me every time is that many of them, like Robert Marchand, start something new at a relatively late age. In 2015, pianist and cancer survivor Harriet Thompson of San Diego, California, at the age of 92, became the oldest woman in the world to complete a marathon. She first resolved to run in a marathon when she was 76. Since then, she has participated in marathons to raise more than $100,000 for the Leukemia and Lymphoma Society. In an interview after one race, she said, "I think that if I can do it, anyone can do it. I've never received training in running even once."

When you hear stories of such old but strong people, hesitation or excuses may pop into your head. My reason for introducing these individuals is not to suggest that we exercise professionally as they do, challenging ourselves to take part in competitions or pushing our physical condition to the limits. My intention is to give you hope and to suggest that we have plenty of potential to live vital, healthy, lives at any age, depending on how we take care of ourselves. Of course, aging is a natural phenomenon that no one can avoid. As you get older, the vigor and functions of your body may decline, and you may develop diseases large and small. But you have a choice. Will you just give up and watch as aging and disease come for you, or will you actively manage your health as the master of your body?

I would like to add a word about people who have severe chronic diseases or physical disabilities, not your ordinary situation. Such people may have a relatively low health score. Being unhealthy, though, does not mean that they can't have happiness or peace.

A 61-year-old Japanese woman I know, Yahata Chieko, has suffered with a trembling body due to early-onset Parkinson's Syndrome. She was wobbly when she walked, always bent over and using a cane. She used only the front part of her feet when she walked, so the soles of her feet never completely touched the ground. She seemed to be floating in the air. She put a good deal of effort into improving her condition by training her body at a Body & Brain Yoga center. One day in June 2011, an amazing change happened to Yahata at a retreat program that I led in Japan. Through deep meditation and collaborative energy healing, she was able to walk with the soles of her feet touching the ground. She could dance without using her cane, raising one leg and then the other. The other participants cheered and applauded, and many were deeply moved and shed tears of joy when they saw her dancing.

It was a day of wonder that Yahata says she will never forget. Here is how she described it: "I was able, after 40 years, to stand with the soles of my feet touching the floor. For me, it is truly a miracle! When the soles of my feet touched the ground, a really wonderful feeling of happiness rose up from the bottoms of my feet. I thought, I can be this happy just by walking with the soles of my feet touching the floor! It was truly a happiness that I felt for the first time since I was born. Although some say they are unhappy because they don't have this or that, I think human beings are already plenty happy just by standing with the soles of their feet touching the earth and being able to breathe; and there is no greater happiness than that!" Ordinary walking, which is nothing special to most people, was a great blessing for her, incomparable with anything else in the world.

The more you have experienced the loss of health, the more precious you may consider health to be. Don't keep limiting yourself by saying, "My body is weak," "I have an illness," or "I have a disability." You can't help but change if you move and exercise your body a little, even a very little, every day. The energy of your mind as well as your body changes through the actions you take to overcome your limitations, and you will gradually experience overflowing courage and confidence—"I can do it."

The times when you train your body and overcome your limitations are moments when you encounter your true self and feel with your whole body that you are truly alive. The joy, sense of reward, and happiness that come through little changes are indescribable. That you have a body that you can move, that you have the awareness and willpower to move them, that you still have life energy—these things fill you with gratitude.

You have probably heard the story of *Life Without Limits* author Nick Vujicic, who was born without arms and legs and only two small, deformed feet. He now circles the globe as a motivational speaker. He writes using the two toes on his left side, operates a computer using his toes and heel, and enjoys swimming, fishing, and even golf. "I enjoy my life. I'm happy," he said in a lecture. "I will try 100 times to get up, and if I fail 100 times, if I fail and I give up, will I ever get up? No! If I fail, I'll try again and again. But I want to tell you, it's not the end. I can get the courage to get up again. Like this [getting up]."

A long time ago, I saw on Korean television the story of a man who suffered from stomach disease. He depended on stomach medication that the hospital gave him. There are many steps leading up Namsan, a mountain in the center of Seoul, but this man's disease had left him too weak to walk up these steps. But one day he made up his mind, "I will not live this way any longer." He began developing muscular strength in his arms, legs, and lower back, starting by doing push-ups. Next he practiced handstands. And several years later, something amazing happened: that man, once weak from disease, climbed the steps of Namsan by walking on his hands in a handstand. Reportedly his stomach disease had completely cleared up, and his body had become healthy.

This man used and mastered his body. "I will no longer suffer from a feeble body or stomach disease, nor will I depend on medications; I will fix my body," he resolved, and the power of his choice—the power of his action—made that possible. Could this have happened if he hadn't made that choice and carried through on what he had resolved to do? Health and physical power can't be created for us by someone else. The power to change yourself depends on you.

When you tell people to improve their physical strength,

they generally imagine training with heavy weights and running on a treadmill at a fitness center. So they give up out of fear, without thinking it through, or they are disappointed with themselves for letting their resolve fizzle out just a few days after registering at a fitness center. Is there no way we can exercise in our daily lives without spending several hours doing it? What I suggest is *opportunistic exercise*. As the name suggests, opportunistic exercise is a lifestyle approach that we use to exercise whenever we get the opportunity.

I came to develop opportunistic exercise as I experienced physical changes in my mid-50s. I was a black belt in taekwondo, judo, and hapkido when I was young, and I could exercise for hours without getting tired, but I was no exception to aging. I began to experience the symptoms of declining physical energy, muscle strength, and reflexes, as well as depression and falling ambition. My eyesight worsened, my gums were in bad shape, and I gained weight so that my body was heavy and my knees weren't doing well. Having lived my whole life without knowing what it was to be physically sick, I thought, "Oh, so this is what it means to be old." And I realized, "If I don't do anything about this, there will be nothing left for me but getting weaker."

That really got my attention. I heard a voice telling me that I must change myself. But how could I return my body to its previous vigor? Where should I begin? I was thinking hard about these questions when I started doing One-Minute Exercise and Longevity Walking, which I will explain in detail. In addition to these two, Belly Button Healing is an excellent form of opportunistic exercise that I developed recently. These aren't exercises you have to set aside special time to do; they're opportunistic exercises you can practice often in your daily life.

You might wonder how effective such simple exercises could be, but through my own experience, I can definitely tell you that these exercises really work. My body became lighter, more agile, and more vigorous through opportunistic exercise. Even now, when I'm almost 70 years old, every day I use the wall to do 10 handstand push-ups—lifting my body by bending and straightening my elbows. And when I golf, I send the ball flying farther and more accurately than I did when I was in my 40s.

We need to develop physical power to keep from being controlled by the condition of our bodies. So, I'll now describe three kinds of lifestyle opportunistic exercise for truly mastering your body and providing yourself with good health.

One-Minute Exercise

Having to deal with a busy schedule of reading dozens of reports, meeting numerous people, and giving lectures from dawn to dusk every day, I started doing one-minute exercises because I had no time to go to a fitness center and work out. I couldn't afford to lose a minute of my precious time.

After washing my hands in the bathroom, I do push-ups against the wall. When sitting in a chair and working, I use my fists or fingers to raise and lower my body repeatedly. Or I do bear walking, crawling with my buttocks and knees in the air and my palms and the soles of my feet on the floor.

For One-Minute Exercise, once every hour do a minute of moderate to vigorous exercise that effectively works your muscles and raises your heart rate in a short period of time—such as push-ups, squats, sit-ups, jumping jacks, jumping in place, and bear walking. It's a good idea to set an alarm to go off every hour to remind you. That means you will be doing a minute of exercise about 10 times a day. Doing a moderate to high-intensity workout during those one-minute exercises may cause muscle pain, so when that happens, mix in gentle exercises such as stretching instead of strength training. If you have a physical disability or disease, exercise in a way that's right for the state of your health and body.

There's no reason you have to do just one minute of exercise. You can do it for five minutes or 10 minutes. When you have the time, combining several exercises will double the effects. For example, if you do bear walking after push-ups or squats, your heart will beat hard, you'll be short of breath, your muscles will ache, and your body will sweat. In a short period of time, you'll experience the effects of high-intensity exercise, which increases heart rate, lung capacity, and body temperature and trains muscle strength.

But if conditions aren't right for longer exercise, invest at least one minute. A minute seems like a short time that blows right past without much meaning, but you won't believe how long it feels when you actually do push-ups for a minute. You might even find yourself sitting down, muscles weak, after being unable to go a whole minute. Hold your breath for a minute, and you'll feel just how long a time it is. If you practice making good use of short periods of time through One-Minute Exercise, it will motivate you to use the rest of your time productively and creatively.

You can get tremendous effects through one minute of moderate to high-intensity exercise once an hour. It's widely known that habitually sitting for long periods of time has a negative effect on health. By exercising once an hour, you can correct that habit. According to the journal *Medicine & Science in Sports & Exercise*, people who sit for 23 or more hours a week have a 64 percent higher risk of heart disease than those who sit for less than 11 hours. Studies have shown that reducing the amount of time you spend sitting each day to less than three hours has the effect of extending your life expectancy two years.

If you spend most of your day in a chair or on a sofa, even if you exercise at a fitness center four or five times a week, you will experience the active couch potato effect that comes from sitting for a long time. In old age, people often sit watching TV instead of doing work. Remember—the more time you spend on the sofa holding a remote control, the worse your health becomes.

A former director of NASA's Life Sciences Division and the author of *Sitting Kills, Moving Heals*, Dr. Joan Vernikos, says that the key to good health is being as active as possible all day. This doesn't mean that you have to exercise for several hours, like an athlete. It means you should move your body whenever you get the chance. The more often you move, the better. Ideally, it's best to get up and move your body every 15 minutes. Even simple, ordinary movement is okay. Intermittent movement that breaks up the habit of uninterrupted sitting is important for maximizing quality of life.

Various physical phenomena occur when you exercise. Your heart rate rises, and your blood volume per heartbeat increases to more quickly circulate oxygen to your muscles and eliminate toxins in your cells. Your breathing rate increases, and your lungs expand and contract more frequently to discharge toxins and send more oxygen into your blood.

Changes occur in more than 20 metabolites during exercise, studies show. Some of those substances burn calories, and some help stabilize blood sugar. Secreted during weight training, testosterone increases protein synthesis, suppresses protein damage, activates satellite cells, and stimulates secretion of various anabolic hormones. Additionally, exercise causes bio-chemical changes that strengthen and renew the brain, particularly the areas associated with memory and learning.

Doing moderate to high-intensity exercises causes your body temperature to rise as you sweat. This not only suddenly fills your once-languid body with vigor, but it also tugs on the reins of your mind. Your mind will really wake up and become alert after one minute of exercise—in short, your spirit is focused. That's why your distracting thoughts disappear and your concentration increases; over time, you develop confidence and passion.

An important point of One-Minute Exercise is that exercise needs to be incorporated into daily life, not separated from it.

In other words, life is exercise, and exercise is life. If you do one minute of exercise every hour in your daily life, you encounter Heaven within you and lead a life that reminds you of your wholeness and creativity. In this sense, I also call One-Minute Exercise *Tongchun Living* (a life of communing with Heaven).

We practice Tongchun Living to keep our consciousness awake. Without that, we don't really exist. Though we have consciousness, it is not a living awareness unless it is awake. We practice Tongchun Living every hour to stay awake. Then our habits and constitution change. We change to having a constitution that allows us to take responsibility for our own health, a constitution that lets us create our own happiness and peace.

Thirty-some years ago, during my early days of teaching the mind-body training methods I created, I provided one-on-one instruction to Chairman Juyung Chung, founder of Hyundai, and Chairman Jonghyun Choi, founder of SK Group, both now global corporations. Looking at these men, I felt that there was something different about them. Their constitutions were different from those of others. More than anything else, they worked hard, used their time efficiently, and had uncommon focus. In other words, their character made success unavoidable for them. This was particularly true of Chairman Chung, who had only a primary school education. It wasn't his good academic background or environment that made him successful; it was his lifestyle that was extraordinary.

What's important is changing your lifestyle, the very way you live. Form a constitution and habits in your daily life that can make you healthy. It's obvious that bad habits make your health worse. Life is created by habits. It is difficult to change in a day's time a lifestyle and habits that you have developed over a long period. That's why I'm telling you to end your past habits as you do one minute of exercise once an hour. Think of it as taking the sword of your will and striking down old habits. And you're introducing new habits by constantly repeating new, positive actions.

One-Minute Exercise is about finding time to break out of your habitual pattern and care for your body and yourself. It is an intentional action to focus on yourself, be present, and be mindful. Once you start doing it, you will naturally start to care about other areas of your life as well.

Many changes will come if you do One-Minute Exercise for a month, for two months, for three months. You'll experience physiochemical changes in your body and emotional changes in your mind, and you'll find yourself developing a new lifestyle of moving your body no matter what. We often spend time lethargically, just staring off into space, and we often waste our time in worrisome or distracting thoughts. We can break free of such moments through One-Minute Exercise. When we are stressed, we can change our mood and get rid of stifling energy this way.

As we do one minute of exercise once an hour, we tell our bodies and emotions, "I am the master." Then we can manage our time by using that next hour more productively and creatively. Escaping from the weak and lazy energy of the body and emotions, we can wake up and pay attention. When we manage our physical condition, we end up managing our time, emotions, and goals, and these come together as life management.

One minute of exercise can also be called *one minute of enlightenment*. In traditional Eastern philosophy, enlightenment is the experience of *no-self*, a state in which the ego disappears. To attain that state of no-self, it is generally thought that you have to go through an extremely difficult process of ascetic practice. In the moment you do one minute of exercise, though, you can experience a state of no-self—that is, free of thoughts. Your mind focuses on your body, and all other thoughts disappear.

Try doing push-ups for a minute without resting. Your thoughts will focus on the feelings in your body so that you have no other thoughts at all. Do pointless worries or delicious food come to mind while you're struggling to do your push-ups? Probably not. The best way to simplify your thoughts is to focus your consciousness in your body. When your mind is focused there, your distracting thoughts will turn off. The light shuts off in your head and comes on in your abdominal core. You're making a deep impression on your body once an hour.

Best of all, One-Minute Exercise increases your level of passion. Through passion you can glimpse your will to live your life. How much passion do you have? It's no exaggeration to say that the answer to this question determines a person's life. Maintaining passion isn't easy for older people with nothing much to do during retirement. It's easy for them to think that they are too old to give themselves completely, with passion, to something new. But passion isn't something you develop because you're young or because you have a good environment. Nor should you hope that other people will inspire greater passion within you, or that it will be revived through a better external environment. Passion is something you make and develop yourself.

One-Minute Exercise is an excellent way to increase the level of passion inside you. You can really feel alive through the beating of your racing heart, through the breath filling your lungs, through the strength of your solid muscles aching from the training you've put them through. That is the moment when you increase the temperature of your passion. "From now on, I'll take responsibility for my health. I'll create my life." You erupt with this will, confidence, and passion. Passion is hope. Kindle the fires of your passion through One-Minute Exercise.

I had an app developed to help people adopt One-Minute Exercise as a daily habit. You can learn more about the app and download it for free at 1MinuteChange.com.

Longevity Walking

A mishap led me to develop Longevity Walking. In 2006, the year I turned 56, I hurt my lower back in a horseback riding accident. It happened in Sedona, Arizona, when I was riding up a mountain and the horse suddenly stopped. Normally, I was always busy, running around with meetings, lectures, and business travel. After the accident, though, I was able to take the time—for the first time in a while—to focus completely on my body so that it could recover. One day, I realized that the way I walked had changed. I no longer had the powerful gait of my youth. At some point I had grown accustomed to what we call in Korea the Chairman's Gait, leaning back with my weight loaded in my heels.

That's when I started researching different ways of walking. I cautiously walked one step at a time, changing my posture and angles, learning like a toddler, and I carefully observed how the feelings in my body changed. I also studied the gaits of the people around me. The way older people walked was different from the way younger people walked.

Through that research, Longevity Walking was born. This way of walking involves aligning your feet in parallel, like the number 11, and pressing down through the *yongchun* (the energy point just below the balls of your feet), flexing all the way to the tips of your toes. Walking pleasantly and strongly, loading my weight on the front of my feet, I felt my mood really improving and strength developing in my body. I walked in my room, walked trails, and even walked golf courses using this method. I walked passionately, continuously creating reasons to walk, and found it fascinating.

Perhaps five months after I had made Longevity Walking a habit in my daily life, I suddenly felt my body overflowing with vigor, as when I was young. I was amazingly lighter and more agile. Happy and grateful just to be able to walk on my own two legs, I realized that walking was more than a simple means of movement—it could be a method for promoting health and, furthermore, a way to experience joy. The mindset you have when you walk is extremely important. The faces of busy people who slog along, walking only to get from point A to point B, are full of worry, but the expressions of those who walk joyfully, thinking of it as exercise, are bright and cheerful. I discovered that health, happiness, and peace are not far off, that they can be found in walking.

Longevity Walking is a simple, easy way of walking. That's why everyone had doubts when I first introduced Longevity Walking. "What effect is that going to have?" But those who have experienced it know, for even walking a little can have an amazing effect in a short time. When you listen to people tell of their experience with Longevity Walking, you find that their stories all have something in common.

- I didn't realize the way you walk is so important.
- Walking is so fun and exciting.
- The heavy pain that was in my legs and feet has vanished, and they are lighter now.
- I used to suffer from insomnia, but now I can get deep sleep.
- My complexion has improved, and my body feels lighter.
- I usually become anxious and tense, but I have much more peace of mind now.
- My body has more energy and my head is clearer, so my focus on work has increased.

Altering one thing—the way you walk—can bring great changes.

Most of us walk without thinking of anything in particular. We're not really interested in our gait. No one criticizes us for walking our own way, whatever is comfortable. We don't learn much about walking in school, and we don't worry about the soles of our feet. But our quality of life changes depending on how we take these steps. Instead of just walking because you have to walk, tell yourself, "I'll exercise as I walk," then walking becomes a means of promoting health for long life, a means of creating happiness.

As we lose muscle mass and our skeleton is reshaped when we get older, the way we walk changes. Beyond about age 60, our posture becomes more stooped, and we develop a waddling, bowlegged gait as our knees fail to extend completely. Weakening knees cause the body's center of gravity to rise from the soles of the feet to the lower back. Later, when our lower backs weaken, our shoulders and neck are tense.

Longevity Walking returns us to the pure, healthy gait we had when we were young children. Energetic children put their weight on the front of their feet as they step out, bodies leaning forward as if they are about to topple over. They don't walk slowly with their hands behind their backs, but with a lively step, adventurously going toward whatever lies ahead. To return an old gait to a youthful one, we need to retrain ourselves in how to walk.

Assume the basic posture of Longevity Walking by standing comfortably and focusing on the acupressure points in the soles of your feet called the yongchun. The yongchun point is located in the hollow spot at the bottom of each foot about a third of the way back from the base of the toes. Stand with your awareness in your yongchun points and your toes gripping the ground. Your body will become balanced as your weight is dispersed through the soles of your feet and the tension rises to your knees, hips, and core in your lower abdomen. Continuing, the energy connects to your chest, your neck, and the crown of your head, stimulating your brain. Now try to walk, imagining that your body is connected from your yongchun points to the crown of your head. You can maximize the natural healing power in your body when you activate your energy all the way to the tips of your toes and restore your original life force through yongchun acupressure.

Longevity Walking is different from ordinary walking in that you activate your brain by tensing the soles of your feet. The toes are where nerves connecting to the brain are most concentrated. To properly flex your toes, you really have to press down on your yongchun points and toes together. In Eastern medicine, the yongchun are considered among the body's most important meridian points. The word yongchun contains this meaning: "The ki energy of life in the human body wells up like a spring of water from the ground." The power transmitted to the brain differs depending on how well you press down into your yongchun points and your toes.

If you do a survey of villages around the world with long-lived populations, you'll find that many are in hilly or mountainous regions. Going up and down hills from morning to evening is a way of walking that puts your weight in the front of the feet.

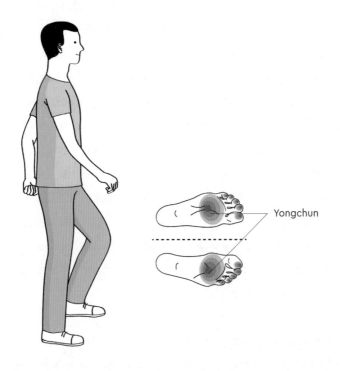

Yongchun

LONGEVITY WALKING
FOR VITALITY AND ENERGY

1. Put your weight in your yongchun energy points.

2. Keep your feet parallel, like the number 11.

3. Press down through your yongchun points and squeeze your toes together.

4. Walk with the feeling of linking the soles of your feet to your brain.

Energy naturally sinks into the soles if you press down on your yongchun points as you walk. The bottoms of your feet grow warmer and your head grows cooler because fire energy that had risen due to stress now sinks into your soles. Keep the head cool and the feet warm—in Eastern medicine, that is said to be the secret of a healthy, long life. The warm energy of fire and the cool energy of water flow together in our bodies. When this balance is unbroken and harmonious—water energy rising upward and remaining cool in the head, fire energy sinking downward and remaining warm in the belly—a body has achieved the *Water Up, Fire Down* state. In this state of circulation, our brains, as well as our bodies, can function maximally. Not only do new energy and vitality well up within us, but our concentration and judgment improve, and our minds become more stable and peaceful.

Most illnesses suffered by modern people result from a reverse flow of energy: the hot energy of the body rises to the head. If this continues, the head becomes hot and thinking is unclear. Concentration drops, and in severe cases it may cause headaches or insomnia. Mental workers who use their heads a lot without moving their bodies need to put even more effort into making Longevity Walking a habit, since a great deal of energy has risen to their heads.

Another point about Longevity Walking is that the feet are kept parallel, like the number 11. Most physically weak or unhealthy people walk with the toes of their feet pointed outward, letting the body's energy slowly leak out. Walking this way for a long time will damage your knees, make your hips go out of alignment, and cause disc or lumbar pain. It also over-works the muscles and bones, causing deformation in the body. But if you walk with your feet parallel, your legs and lower core will tense, and your lower back will straighten. When the spine is straight, energy and blood circulate smoothly and the flow of cerebrospinal fluid improves, resulting in a clearer head.

It's good to tuck your tailbone slightly forward when you do Longevity Walking. When you pull the tailbone area forward just a bit, your anal sphincter muscles contract, allowing energy to collect more readily in your lower belly. Your lower abdomen grows warmer, energy rises along your spine, starting in your tailbone, and the blood and energy circulation of your entire body is enhanced as ki energy accumulates in your core.

Often the first thing that comes to mind for those who are tired and in poor physical condition is that they want to lie down. And as energy decreases with age, people tend to spend more time resting than being active. The more you lie down, though, the weaker your body becomes. You've probably had the experience of feeling wiped out even when you've gotten plenty of sleep on the weekend. That's because you were lying down for a long time without good ki energy circulation. When you get up after sleeping, naturally your body feels unrespon-sive, without energy. If you really want to lie down, do so after getting your blood and energy circulation going by doing Lon-gevity Walking for five or 10 minutes. Then you'll be able to get a deep sleep and wake up refreshed.

Some 2,500 years ago, Hippocrates said, "Walking is man's best medicine." Walking is a whole-body exercise that mobilizes all 600-plus muscles that make up our bodies and the 200-plus bones that move with them. In particular, it stimulates the many nerves stretching out through the soles of the feet and promotes active blood circulation and metabolism in the legs, playing an important role in training the muscles in the lower body and helping to prevent aging.

Walking is a way to effectively supply oxygen to the brain. Although accounting for only about 2 percent of body weight, the brain is the body part that uses the most energy. It uses 15 percent of the blood leaving the heart and about 25 percent of the oxygen that enters the body through breathing, even during rest. If the blood supply to the brain is interrupted for about 15 seconds, a person loses consciousness; at four minutes, brain cells suffer irreparable damage. When brain cell activity drops, the head is unclear, concentration declines, and ambition fades. Blood circulation must be smooth if enough oxygen is to be supplied to the brain. By moving your legs—the so-called second heart—you can assist the movement of your heart. This facilitates blood circulation, resulting in good oxygen supply and enabling you to remain in good health from the top of your head to the tips of your toes.

Walking not only delays brain-related aging, like shrinkage in brain size and functional decline, but it can also increase brain size. Dr. Kirk I. Erickson of the University of Pittsburgh discovered an increase of 2 percent in the size of the hippocampus, which governs memory, in people between the ages of 60 and 80 who walked 30 to 45 minutes a day, three days a week, for a year. Conversely, if we don't use our bodies, their functions are bound to decline. As one example, if you injure one leg and wear a cast for a while, you will see when you take it off that the healed leg has become thinner than the other leg. One test studied how muscles atrophied in strong, healthy males when they spent three weeks lying down without moving. While the muscles of their arms stayed the same, their leg muscles became some 15 percent thinner. With nine weeks of training, the atrophied leg muscles returned to their original condition. Such studies appear to demonstrate scientifically that our legs atrophy first unless we walk. Also, people must spend three times as much time rebuilding muscle as it took to lose the muscle.

Busy legs, it is said, make for a long life. Our legs are our source of vitality. The vitality of the human body depends on how well we maintain our muscles, and some 30 percent of our muscle is in our legs—or more than 40 percent for athletes. The more muscle you have in your legs, the more energetic you are. Conversely, the less muscle you have, the less energy you have. Elderly people easily suffer fractures because they have lost muscle mass. Rather than blaming your age if your legs shake after climbing a few stairs, start daily training for developing leg strength right now.

You can promote health in your daily life simply and naturally through Longevity Walking. And you automatically become happier and more peaceful when you are physically healthier. You're more generous to those around you, and you develop a desire to help them. This is why I find poor health to be the starting point of all problems.

Seongcheol Moon, a 65-year-old orthopedist who has worked on South Korea's Jeju Island for more than 35 years, believes that Longevity Walking rapidly alleviates pain in the musculoskeletal system of his patients by correcting skeletal imbalance. He has seen many patients with skeletal abnormalities caused by their professions. While using Longevity Walking in his treatment, he has seen many patients experience improvements in knee pain, hip pain, lumbar pain, cervical and shoulder pain, and headaches due to the resulting spinal realignment.

A typical example is his own wife. She had suffered for more than two decades with weak bones and genetically weak knee joints. She was also a doctor, so she first attempted all the treatments of modern medicine. If they were effective, Dr. Moon would apply them to his patients. However, none of the treatments were fully able to relieve her intermittent joint edema and pain. Walking and other forms of exercise caused severe knee pain, which made it difficult for her to continue exercising, so Dr. Moon had to listen to his wife's criticism of him as "an orthopedist who can't even fix his own wife's legs."

After learning Longevity Walking from me, he started spending an hour a day walking with his wife on a mountain near his clinic. They went for short walks at first and gradually increased their walking distance. They walked a little slowly in the beginning so they could be conscious of their yongchun points and really get the feeling of their connection to their brains. Previously, Dr. Moon's wife had focused her awareness on her painful knees when she walked. But she said that her consciousness moved to the soles of her feet and her brain as she did Longevity Walking, and her whole body seemed to stand upright. After about a month, she no longer had any pain, her physical activity had increased, her body fat had decreased, and she had developed confidence about her knee pain. They were able to climb up Mt. Halla, the highest mountain in South Korea, which would have been unimaginable before.

Based on his wife's experience, Dr. Moon now teaches and recommends daily Longevity Walking to his patients. Even patients who initially didn't want to walk because of their pain say that their bodies grew stronger and the pain decreased as they gradually increased their time walking with proper posture. Although there are many approaches to correct walking, Dr. Moon recommends Longevity Walking as highly effective for quickly relaxing physical tension, correcting physical imbalance, and alleviating chronic pain.

I have developed an in-depth Longevity Walking guide with step-by-step instructions and illustrations for people who are interested in this method. You can download it at Live120YearsBook.com.

Belly Button Healing

As a third form of opportunistic exercise for protecting your health, I suggest Belly Button Healing. This is a method of self-healing that promotes the health of body and mind by stimulating the belly button, which is considered a kind of trigger point. I have developed numerous mind-body health practices over the last 37 years, but I have always wanted to find easier and more powerful methods. Belly Button Healing is as simple as Longevity Walking, but the area of the body stimulated is so unusual that people are often surprised and ask, "What did you just say?" After experiencing Belly Button Healing directly, they are again surprised by the power and effectiveness of these simple movements.

The basic idea of Belly Button Healing is to rhythmically and repeatedly compress the belly button, as I will explain. Improvements felt by those who have experienced Belly Button Healing include good digestion, better sleep, improved mood, enhanced energy, and pain relief. Why does this simple motion have such a variety of effects? The answer lies in the location of the belly button. The navel is in the center of the human body, the center of the abdomen. Gathered around the belly button are all the major organs for maintaining life, including the digestive, circulatory, respiratory, and immune organs. Promoting good digestion, facilitating blood circulation, breathing deeply, and strengthening the immune system are essential components of good health. The button that turns these on all at once is the belly button.

Of course, to really understand Belly Button Healing, you need to experience it directly. Start by lying comfortably on your back. A seated posture is also acceptable if you can't lie down at the moment. Relax your body and mind, and really try to feel the condition of your body—your breathing rhythm, your sense of vitality, and the temperature of your belly and legs. Now bring together the tips of your index, middle, and ring fingers on both hands and use them to press your navel repeatedly. Do this through the clothes you're wearing, not directly on your skin. Close your eyes and concentrate your awareness on your belly button, pressing it rhythmically about 100 times per minute. You can increase the number of repetitions as you get used to the exercise. There is also a special tool called Healing Life that I developed for doing Belly Button Healing effectively, which you can use if you have it.

If you have a constricted feeling in your chest, exhale naturally through your nose or mouth to discharge the stagnant air and energy in your chest. Stop your belly button presses after about 100 to 300 repetitions.

While in a comfortable posture, close your eyes and breathe, concentrating on your belly button and lower abdomen to begin Belly Button Breathing. The basic process is simple. To maximize the effects of Belly Button Breathing, however, you must add your imagination to this exercise. Visualize that there is a breathing hole in your belly button, as if the nose on your face has moved to your navel. When you breathe in, push your belly out and visualize life energy entering and filling it through the "nose" of your navel. When you breathe out, concentrate your awareness in your navel as you contract your belly, pulling it toward your back. Imagine that the energy of life is being injected into your abdomen through your navel as you visualize your belly repeatedly inflating and deflating like a rubber balloon.

As your breathing grows deeper and more comfortable, you

will feel as if you are being supplied with life energy, as you were through your umbilical cord in your mother's womb, as if you were going back to that infinitely comfortable and peaceful time when you were receiving the love of your mother in that safe, cozy place. Instead of feeling that you are a separate organism, you have a sense of stability and unity, of being connected with your mother through your belly button.

After no more than about five minutes of this, your breathing will deepen and become more natural, your abdomen and even your lower body will grow warmer, and your head will become clearer. You will be charged with vital energy, becoming more relaxed at the same time. So many positive effects in such a short time—isn't that amazing?

The most direct effect of Belly Button Healing is intestinal health improvement. In addition to handling the digestion of food, absorption of nutrients, and excretion of waste from our bodies, our intestines are deeply involved in detoxification and immunity. Recent studies on intestinal microbiota and intestinal and brain condition have also revealed that our gut is closely associated with our emotions and thinking.

The organ stimulated most directly through Belly Button Healing is the small intestine, located immediately below the belly button. Rhythmically and regularly pressing the belly button activates the peristalsis of the small intestine muscle, aiding digestion and making bowel movements regular and smooth. About 30 to 40 percent of your body's entire blood volume flows through the abdominal organs. By pressing and stimulating your belly button, you can effectively increase

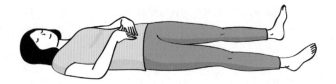

BELLY BUTTON HEALING

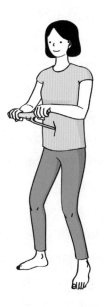

1. You can do Belly Button Healing lying down or standing up.

2. Relax your body and breathe comfortably for about one minute while focusing on your lower abdomen.

3. Press your belly button with the three middle fingertips of both hands rhythmically, repeatedly, and mindfully for about 100 to 300 repetitions.

4. After finishing, spend a couple of minutes focusing on your breathing, feeling your body more relaxed and refreshed.

 You can use a Belly Button Healing wand, a tool specially designed for the practice, for easier and more effective application.

blood circulation in your abdomen, facilitating the supply of oxygen and nutrients to your whole body. While healthy eating habits are fundamental for the health of the intestines, Belly Button Healing has the great advantage of being able to contribute substantially to gut health through a simple exercise, even without food or medication.

Additionally, the abdominal lymph nodes are concentrated around the belly button. Lymph nodes are organs of the immune system. Belly Button Healing assists immune reaction and excretion of waste products by appropriately stimulating these lymph nodes to facilitate the flow of lymphatic fluid.

Researchers are becoming increasingly aware of the importance of the immune function of intestinal microorganisms. Three hundred to 1,000 species of microbes live in the intestines, an environment referred to as gut microbiota. Gut microbes not only break down food and create vitamins and hormones, but they also stop pathogens. The enteric immune system, which includes the activity of immune cells and microbes in the gut, accounts for 70 to 80 percent of the body's immunity. Belly Button Healing helps you improve your gut environment and increase your abdominal temperature by exercising the gut and promoting blood and oxygen circulation in the intestines, resulting in enhanced immunity.

As it turns out, science has discovered that the neurons that manage your gut from esophagus to anus, the enteric nervous system (ENS), can operate independently from your brain. Like your brain, the ENS has cells that take in information, cells that process it, and cells that tell your digestive system what to do.

Even if the connection between the enteric nervous system and the brain is cut off or the brain stops working, the ENS can keep doing its job. That's why the ENS and its related cells are called the second brain or the gut brain.

While the brain in your head contains about 100 billion cells, the gut brain has about 300 to 500 million—about five times the number in the spinal cord. The function of our gut is so important that it has a direct line to the brain via a cranial nerve called the vagus nerve. More than 2,000 neural fibers connect our head brain with our gut brain, allowing the two brains to communicate closely and rapidly. That's why when a problem develops in the intestines, it affects the brain immediately; conversely, when a problem develops in the brain, problems develop in the intestines. Have you ever had a stomachache when you heard bad news or were nervous? Have you ever had a headache when you had gas or constipation? This shows the tight connection between the intestines and the brain.

The influence of our gut brain on our head brain goes even deeper. For example, the neurons and hormone-producing cells in the gut generate chemical signals that affect our emotions. Approximately 50 percent of our dopamine, the neurotransmitter that lets us feel pleasure and reward, is created in the gut brain. More than 95 percent of our serotonin, the neurotransmitter that gives us feelings of happiness and well-being, is also created in the gut, while only 3 percent is made in the brain.

Serotonin and dopamine affect mood, motivation, sleep, sexual desire and function, memory and learning, and social behavior. Depression and anxiety, which develop when we don't have enough serotonin or dopamine, may be strongly influenced by problems in the intestines. Improving intestinal health can increase serotonin and dopamine secretion, enabling us to maintain a positive mood and to feel satisfied and motivated. Most children with conditions such as autism or ADHD (attention deficit hyperactivity disorder) have issues with their gut. Some adult brain conditions, such as Alzheimer's disease, have also been found to have a strong correlation with gut condition.

Studies have shown that people over 50 with symptoms of depression caused by a lack of serotonin are twice as likely to develop vascular dementia as those the same age without depression, and they're 65 percent more likely to develop Alzheimer's. Many of these brain conditions have improved when gut conditions improved—and sometimes this has been more effective than traditional treatments that target the brain directly.

I've done several conferences with Dr. Emeran Mayer, world-famous gut-brain health researcher and author of *The Mind-Gut Connection*, so I've had the opportunity to talk with him about a holistic perspective for gut-brain health. He says that the solar plexus chakra, which is near the belly button, is traditionally thought to control an individual's energy, fear, and anxiety, as well as the digestion of food, and that this suggests a connection between the gut and the brain. He says that activating the solar plexus chakra by direct physical stimulation, as in Belly Button Healing, massage, or indirect stimulation as in yoga or abdominal breathing, can lead to enhanced gut-brain connectivity.

As mentioned previously, our guts and brains are connected by the vagus nerve. This nerve extends from the brainstem to virtually all organs in the body, including the small intestine, stomach, liver, kidneys, lungs, and heart. The vagus nerve acts as a two-way information superhighway, delivering to the organs the brain's commands for regulating breathing, heartbeat, and so on, and delivering to the brain information about each organ, including whether the stomach and other digestive organs are empty.

The belly button is the most effective point for directly stimulating the vagus nerve from outside the body because it has few layers of muscle beneath it. Repeatedly and rhythmically pressing the belly button stimulates the vagus nerve in the small intestine, and that can have a ripple effect on the brain and other organs.

The greatest benefit is an increased ability to control stress. The vagus nerve is the body's largest parasympathetic nerve. Parasympathetic nerves cause our bodies to rest, supplement our energy through digestion, discharge toxins, and repair damage. Conversely, sympathetic nerves cause a stress reaction that excites and tenses the body. If the sympathetic nerves are overactivated, we end up suffering all kinds of disorders—hypertension, diabetes, heart disease, arteriosclerosis, perceptual dysfunction, indigestion. That's why stress is considered the source of many diseases. Belly Button Healing stimulates the parasympathetic nerves, deeply resting and relaxing our bodies. Saliva pools in the mouth, and breathing becomes deeper after just five minutes of Belly Button Healing, evidence that the parasympathetic nervous system has been activated and is boosting the body's natural healing power.

The Korean name for this navel energy point is *shingwol*, or "palace of God," the place where God comes and goes and dwells. According to Eastern medicine, stimulating the shingwol point improves the body's immunity and facilitates the flow of energy and blood in the abdominal organs, warming the body and restoring overall health. The shingwol energy point is used for emergency treatment when someone suddenly loses consciousness or collapses from high blood pressure or stroke, as well as for treating intestinal diseases that result from low body temperature, cold limbs, or women's reproductive issues such as menstrual disorders and infertility.

Belly Button Healing is a simple, effective health practice for seniors whose energy is weak and whose breathing is gradually becoming shallower. By compressing the abdomen, it is possible to pump the blood collecting in the intestines and circulate it throughout the body. This also exercises the abdominal muscles and makes the intestines flexible, allowing the diaphragm to sink deeply into the abdomen. When you lack vitality or you're tired, press your belly button for even one minute and then do Belly Button Breathing; you will soon feel your body recovering vigor and growing warmer.

It's a little like using CPR on someone whose heart has stopped. Belly Button Healing, we might say, is energy CPR for reviving the vitality of someone whose health has collapsed.

In the United States, many who have directly experienced its powerful effects are volunteering for Project Revitalize, visiting assisted living facilities in their communities and teaching Belly Button Healing to seniors and staff members.

Deep breathing is the key to maintaining health, vitality, stability, and peace of mind in old age. People tend to take shorter breaths as they get older. When they are babies, they breathe deeply with their lower abdomen. But as time passes, their vitality decreases and the energy in their chest is blocked by stress, making their breathing shallow and causing them to do chest breathing. Before meeting death, their breathing is very shallow and centered in the throat, until they can breathe no more. For older people, there is nothing more effective than Belly Button Breathing for recovering deep, natural breathing in a short period of time. You can also learn to breathe deeply through a method called Breathing Meditation, described in detail in Chapter 10.

Belly Button Healing can also be used to find pain points in and around your navel and then press on those spots to resolve problems in associated parts of the body. The goal of repeatedly compressing the belly button and then breathing is to enhance vitality. Pressing on the pain points around the navel is effective for releasing energy that has stagnated in the abdomen, nearby organs, shoulders, lower back, and hip joints. This could be called a kind of belly button reflexology.

Lemuel Carlos, an immigration lawyer in his late 40s, lives in Phoenix, Arizona. His family is well known in the Filipino community of Phoenix for their business and nonprofit activities. He learned about Belly Button Healing through the Body & Brain Yoga center he attended, but at first he had no intention of trying it. "That's weird," he thought.

His thinking changed when his father's health greatly improved through Belly Button Healing. His father, now 81 years old, had a kidney transplant 23 years ago. He got along well until his kidneys rapidly deteriorated about a year ago and he ended up on long-term dialysis. But after starting Belly Button Healing and yoga, his health greatly improved; his creatinine levels, which had risen to 5.1, dropped to 2.3 in a few months. He went to the hospital less often, his appetite returned, and his diabetes and blood pressure returned to normal.

Motivated by his father's experience, Lemuel began doing Belly Button Healing himself. Dealing with legal problems related to immigration and divorce in his law practice causes him a lot of stress, and that was greatly reduced when he started Belly Button Healing. He says that five minutes of Belly Button Healing has the same effect for him as walking for about 15 to 20 minutes.

Doing Belly Button Healing when he's tired and his concentration has dropped wakes him up, he says, and is much better than drinking coffee. After he had surgery for a tumor on his spine 25 years ago, raising his left arm felt unnatural. After doing Belly Button Healing for several months, he no longer feels any discomfort. Many people in his Filipino community run assisted living businesses, and he is actively telling them about Belly Button Healing. He also recommends it to clients.

If you would like to learn more about this practice, please

see my book *Belly Button Healing: Unlocking Your Second Brain for a Healthy Life* or visit BellyButtonHealing.com.

Master Mind, Master Body

Managing your physical condition is essential for living a life of completion, one that provides true inner satisfaction in the second half of your life. Make exercise a part of your life, keeping in mind that health is the cornerstone upon which you can build your quality of life in old age, making possible the life you want.

You are fortunate if you already have a habit of regular exercise. If you don't yet have that habit, start developing it now. Move your body every chance you get, choosing exercises that are right for your condition and situation, using the exercises introduced in this book—One-Minute Exercise, Longevity Walking, Belly Button Healing. And always remember: you can master your mind once you have mastered your body.

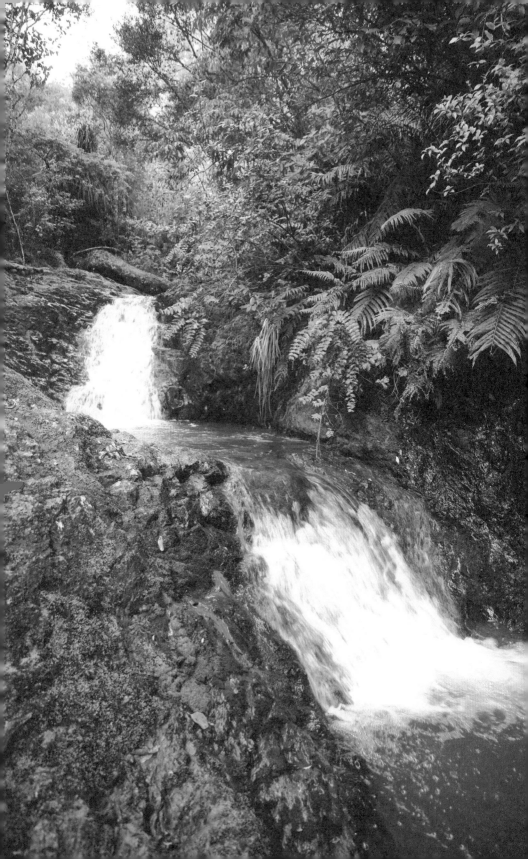

CHAPTER 6

Discover New Sources of Happiness

J ust as everybody wants to be healthy, everyone wants to be happy. But more and more people seem to feel that they are *not* happy. People, especially as they get older, are experiencing deeper and more frequent forms of unhappiness in many spheres of life: chronic illnesses, alienation or disruption of personal relationships, weakening of economic power. Suddenly facing their social roles greatly reduced during retirement, people are likely to find their self-esteem withering away.

What about you? Are you happy? As you read this book, you will probably have a serious longing to be happier and live more fully in the second half of your life. To give yourself the opportunity to satisfy that thirst, you must have the courage to ask yourself some important questions.

- Am I happy now?
- When, specifically, do I feel happy?
- Do I feel happy when someone else makes me happy?
- Do I tend to feel that it's my external environment that is keeping me from being happy?

- Do I consider inner happiness important?
- Do I tend to act proactively to create inner happiness?

If you feel happy now and are actively working to be even happier, that's great. But if you are unhappy now and worried about why, then you urgently need to find the cause.

Master Your Environment

As I've met people from all walks of life and helped them to live more satisfying lives, I've found that there have been two main reasons that people feel they are unhappy.

First, they are unsatisfied with the environment they face. In other words, they consider themselves unhappy because they lack something. Environment refers not only to the situations surrounding you, such as your economic power and personal relationships, but also to all the situations you face, even including your physical and mental health. Some people think they are unhappy because they're not physically well, while others think they are unhappy because they don't have enough money. Others think they are unhappy because they don't have a partner or friends with whom to share their hearts. These things are all part of the environment surrounding you.

If you let environmental factors determine your happiness or unhappiness, it will be difficult to avoid being a slave to your environment all your life. To be happy, you would have to wait for your environment to change. Instead, you should become the master of your environment, leading it and causing it to change instead of blaming it for your unhappiness. Without this attitude, you'll fail to make use of even a good environment and will instead be controlled by it. Many people, though they have wealth and power, become mired in a hell of unhappiness because they misuse these things.

When you get older, the first thing you really experience is changes in your physical environment. You are weaker, your skin loses its elasticity, and you get sick more frequently. Such physical changes often are accompanied by uncomfortable emotions such as anxiety, sadness, and fear. How can we deal with such emotions? One powerful method is to move your awareness to your body through such things as opportunistic exercise, which I talked about in the previous chapter. If you practice this regularly, you'll develop a sense for extricating yourself from negative emotions and for improving your mood quickly in any situation.

You must understand the relationship between yourself and your emotions: emotions are not you, but yours. Emotions are merely a variable environment that affects you like any other surrounding that you experience. You can choose to walk away from an emotion the same way you walk out of a room. You can change your emotions because they are only your internal environment, not the essence of who you are.

No matter how much you try to control your mind through training and meditation, however, negative emotions will arise within you. You'll be lonely, sad, or angry at times. That is normal. As long as we live entangled with countless people and events, such emotions will arise. Because we live in many external and internal environments, emotions are bound to arise according to changes in those environments—just as our days are not always sunny but sometimes cloudy, windy, or rainy. Holding your center allows you to calmly watch such changes.

Negative emotions—like loneliness, sadness, anger, and fear—are not necessarily bad. If we couldn't feel anxiety or fear, how would humanity have been able to survive this long, dealing with life-threatening crises? How boring, dull, and shallow would our lives be if sadness and anger disappeared from them altogether? Our moments of joy and happiness feel that much more beautiful and precious because we have trying moments, too.

It's important not to get bogged down by negative emotions. It's natural for emotions to arise, but you must guard against getting stuck in those feelings and being led around by them. Flailing about in a quicksand of negative emotions for a long time saps your strength and makes you feel lonely, afraid, and unhappy. Such emotions bring your energy down, making it darker and heavier. In particular, once you're stuck in negative feelings about getting older, depressing thoughts come one after another, tempting you to give up. We begin to tell ourselves, "I'm powerless, sick, bored, lonely, and gradually getting older. I could die at any time. I'm scared."

To avoid getting stuck in negative emotions, you need to be aware of your emotional state and to develop the strength to escape from it. That is the power of the soul. Nothing but the brightness of consciousness, the power of the soul, can calm the rolling waves of emotion. Once the power of your soul is awake, you can watch your feelings transform and renew your consciousness. And you become able to *use* your environment as you wish instead of being controlled by it. You think of your environment, whether good or difficult, as a problem that has been given to you for the growth of your soul, and you explore ways to achieve your soul's growth through it. Will you get stuck in your environment, becoming its slave, or will you master your environment, putting it to good use? You must choose. Only then can you create happiness and become the true master of your life.

Looking back on my own life, I realize that I've suffered many twists and turns, and many struggles. Those difficult environments actually trained me. There were so many difficulties that I can't list them all here, but I'll tell you about one experience that put me in a very embarrassing environment.

It happened about 20 years ago when I came from South Korea to the United States to start teaching Body & Brain Yoga, the mind and body training method that I developed. I boarded the plane with great hope and expectation, crossed the Pacific Ocean, passed over the American continent, and then finally arrived at JFK International Airport in New York City. I had collected my bag and loaded it on a cart, and I was walking to meet the person who was supposed to pick me up. That's when someone suddenly came up and started talking to me. I didn't understand a word he was saying because I couldn't speak English well. He got right in my face and was going on and on about something. I had the feeling that he was asking me for directions, but I didn't know the area and couldn't explain that to him, so I could only stand there looking frustrated.

I got a weird feeling, though. If I couldn't answer him, he should have asked someone else. But there he was, continually smiling and trying to use body language. I thought, "Wait a minute!" Then I turned around and saw someone else taking off with my bag. I looked back the other way, but the person who'd been speaking to me was already gone. Only then did I realize, "Oh, man, I've had my bag stolen." The bag contained the uniform I was going to wear when teaching classes, my books, and $5,000 in seed money. I met up with the person who'd come to get me and filed a report with the police, but I had no way of recovering my bag.

How would you have felt in that situation? As you can imagine, I was upset. "How could something like this happen as soon as I arrived in the land of America? Did I make a mistake in coming here? Is this a bad omen for my future? Should I go back to Korea?" All kinds of negative thoughts came to mind. I couldn't go back to Korea because of that, though. "I'll pioneer the work in America," I had told my students in Korea when I left. "You all handle things in Korea." So I couldn't even think of going back. It was also difficult for me to tell anyone that my bag had been stolen. It seemed to me that people would whisper, "An enlightened Tao master got his money stolen? Shouldn't he be able to just look at someone and know that he was a thief?"

I had come full of hope, but in an instant I had fallen into despair. It seemed like it would be hard to begin my activity in America with such an unpleasant feeling. Emotion is a kind of energy that affects the energy of the mind and body, so I was not starting off well. With that kind of energy, I felt like I didn't have the strength I would need to start such an enormous task. I might have been justified in giving up right then and there, but fortunately I already knew I didn't have to stay in that state. I realized I had to put myself in a new mood somehow, even though problems just kept developing.

So, I decided to find a positive message I could give myself. I thought about what it might mean that I lost my bag as soon as I came to America. And this message came to mind: "I haven't lost a bag and money. I came to America and donated $5,000 to New York. That guy's situation must've been pretty bad for him to have taken the money." I felt a little better after changing my thinking in this way. "I've donated $5,000, so I will be blessed in the future. A thousandfold blessing will come back to me within 10 years," I said, giving myself a concrete message.

My mood really improved after I thought about it in this way, and an unstoppable ambition welled up within me. Nothing in my external environment had changed. Only one thing had changed: my thinking. All I did was change my thinking about one thing, but I gained the strength to face reality with an attitude that was 180 degrees opposite of what it had been. And the future I had hoped for really did become a reality 10 years later. Changing your ideas, giving your brain a good message—this is a first step that can change your environment.

We all encounter obstacles great and small as we live our lives. Reactions differ from person to person, though, even for the same obstacle. Some are blocked and make no further progress, while others boldly break through and continue on their way. The individual who has successfully dealt with a setback has experienced that opportunities and blessings are waiting beyond it. Obstacles are there to be overcome; we are trained and grow stronger in the process of overcoming them. Don't fear obstructions. It's difficult to break through a barrier if you think it is a thick wall. Based on the experiences of my life so far, obstacles are not thick walls; they are merely thin paper curtains that look thick on the outside. Push through, and they open up. Many people, though, are afraid and don't even think about breaking through those walls.

When an obstacle appears, when you're faced with a difficult situation, don't give up in despair. First try to think that there is a reason for everything in the environment you're facing. And try switching to the idea that it's an environment capable of developing the power of your soul. With such a mindset, you can see everything as something to be studied, as grist for the mill of your growth. And you become capable of changing the environment, as the creator standing at its center. Then you can live your life not waiting for happiness to come from the outside, but creating and sharing happiness yourself.

The first reason many people feel unhappy is that they are dissatisfied with the environment they face. Perhaps they didn't get the opportunities they wanted, suffered from poor family relations, or faced financial difficulties their whole life. Would they have been happier if they had spent their time in a good environment, if none of those troubles had been present? Not necessarily, which is something you have probably seen for yourself, directly or indirectly. Many of those who have plenty of wealth and power, those who have grasped success, including popular celebrities, consider themselves unhappy. Even with a good house, car, and partner—commonly thought to be conditions for happiness—tedium and boredom are bound to come. Why? They have failed to discover something granting them true meaning and motivation in life, something that allows them to live every day with heart-pounding passion. This lack of a sense of purpose is the second reason people feel they are not happy.

After we retire, we have an incredible amount of time to use as we want until we die, but all that time feels overwhelming, and we don't know how in the world to spend it. Assuming that you will live 35 years after retiring and you have eight hours a day to engage in meaningful activity, that comes to about 100,000 productive hours. How will you use 100,000 hours in a way that's substantial and rewarding? If you spend monotonous days in old age eating good food in a good house without much happening every day for decades, could we call that a truly meaningful, happy life? Is there no way to live our lives so that when we close our eyes on our final day, we can say, "I really lived a good life. I feel fulfilled and really proud of myself"?

There is. It means transforming our ideas about happiness. And it means discovering new sources of happiness.

Another word for happiness is *joy*. There are different kinds of joy. Basically, there are joys that come from satisfying instinctual desires, like the joy of eating and the joy obtained through sex. On the next level are two kinds of joy—one that comes from possession and one that comes from control. Up to this point, we're talking about joys that animals also feel. These joys are deeply associated with the lower dahnjon or lower chakras, which generally control the energies of the body and desire.

In youth, desires for food, sex, possession, and control are powerful. But continuing to cling only to these joys when you're older will bring misfortune upon yourself. I'm not suggesting that you shouldn't pursue such joys any longer. You can still enjoy food and sex, and you can exercise ownership and control through economic activities. However, if you seek to relieve your boredom only through the joys that come from indulging and satisfying such desires, a meaningful life and true happiness will gradually grow more distant.

Old age is a time to find new sources of happiness. Instead of being attached only to the joys that come from the desires you sought to satisfy in the past, discover joys of a higher level. It's like digging a new well. If the spring waters you used to drink no longer relieve your thirst, you need to dig another well. Don't just stand there watching the old well dry up, hoping for the rains or someone else to come along and refill it for you. There are many other sources of happiness; if you're willing, you can dig another well. Old age is a time to seriously focus on finding the happiness that springs up from within, not the happiness that comes from external things such as wealth and power. The inner spring of happiness never runs dry, and it offers truly pure water that can quench the thirst of souls weary of a tedious, mundane life.

Fortunately, a system in our bodies makes it impossible *not* to pursue higher-level joy in our old age. Appetite and libido decline naturally with age, and hormonal changes reshape our physical desires. These needs still exist, of course, but they are much reduced compared with the peak of youth. Like a caterpillar that no longer eats but spends its time transforming in its cocoon, in old age we humans experience a decline in appetite, are much less bound by our sexual needs, and have more time for solitary contemplation.

Like caterpillars that prepare to transform into butterflies to soar in the sky, we humans raise our eyes from the ground and look toward the heavens. We reflect on how we have lived our lives and think hard about how we will find closure before passing away. In this way, naturally pursuing a higher level of joy in old age is a principle of the human body and a principle of nature. That's why selfish people who are still obsessed with their desires even into old age seem ugly. Going with the changes in your body is living according to the natural order.

Although there are different kinds of high-level joy we can pursue in the second half of our lives, three of them give us true inner satisfaction and lead us to a life of completion. The first is the joy of *Hongik*—a Korean word that means living for the good of all, which involves working for the benefit of others. The second is the joy of awakening, and the third is the joy of creation. These three kinds of joy are deeply related to the stages of development of the energy centers in our bodies. The joy you feel when you have great, pure, unconditional love, when you practice Hongik, is felt when the energy of the middle dahnjon in the heart is activated. The joy of awakening and the joy of creation are felt when the energy of the upper dahnjon in the head is activated.

The Joy of Hongik

When do you feel happy? Many people say they feel happy when they love and are loved by someone else. When asked when they feel unhappy, they say it is when they don't give and receive love. Love is definitely a bizarre emotion, the understanding of which seems just beyond our reach. Love can cause us to float on clouds of happiness at one moment and then, suddenly, send us tumbling headlong into hellish misery. To understand the essence of love, we have to ask where it comes from.

Not all love is on the same level. If we divide love into two general categories, one is emotional love that seeks to possess and control, while the other is the pure, unconditional love of the soul. These two energies of love are mixed in the heart— the middle dahnjon—but their roots are different. Emotional love is affected by energy rising from the lower dahnjon. The energy of sexual desire, the energy of the desire to possess and control, rises to create emotional energy in the chest. People commonly call the feelings that stem from such desires love, but they could also be delusion, attachment, or greed.

Pure, unconditional love doesn't seek to possess, and it doesn't seek to control. The reason love turns into unhappiness at some moment is that it seeks to possess and control. When your love is about to change into unhappiness, check whether you're seeking to possess and control the other person—although, of course, the other person might be at fault, too. Set aside such attachments and choose the pure love of the soul instead.

The happiness of those who have an emotional kind of love is generally determined by the reaction of the other person. They're happy if the other person loves them, unhappy if they don't. Conversely, the happiness of those who have the pure love of the soul is centered within themselves. They feel true happiness as they share the pure love in their hearts. They focus on loving others instead of trying to draw the energy of love from others. They don't expect or calculate that something will come back to them in exchange for loving the other person. They believe in the soul and in the bright, true nature of the other person and try to develop it instead of trap the other person in a mold, assessing and judging them.

That is true love and compassion.

This ideal love is the sort that should be pursued in old age. Rather than possessing and controlling one another, older couples can teach and learn from their partners. They can be soulmates and fellow travelers who walk the path of life together, contributing to each other's spiritual growth. Then they'll have subtler but greater happiness in their golden years.

This love of the soul isn't limited to couples. Many people who have been separated from their spouses by death or divorce have great trouble enduring their loneliness. But if you feel that you won't be happy until you have a partner, you're digging a well of unhappiness. There's nothing that says you must give the energy of love in your heart to just one person. When we look around, we find many people who need our love and help. That's why many enlightened elders choose to volunteer or to contribute their talents to their neighbors or communities.

You feel incredible joy when you love and accept others unconditionally, when you share what you have without calculating your own interests, when you sacrifice yourself for others out of what arises in your heart. When you share your energy of pure love, you discover a wellspring of joy you haven't been able to feel any other way.

A life of helping others, Hongik, is the founding ideology and educational philosophy of Korea. *Hong* means widely, and *ik* means to benefit, so it means that a Hongik person works for the good of many people, not just for themselves and their families. If we say that loving one person is small love, then Hongik is big love.

Some people have a lot of love in their hearts, but they keep it locked up there without sharing its energy with others, which leads to their unhappiness. They really want to use their energy of love, but they're failing to do so. Moreover, those who have been hurt by small love may close their hearts because they distrust others. Even small love is beautiful and meaningful if it involves a relationship of mutual respect and care. When mature, small love acts as a signpost leading us to big love. But you bring unhappiness on yourself if, obsessed only with small love, you wait for love to find you. Our hearts are truly happy, free, and peaceful when we have big love. Then our soul's energy grows and becomes more powerful. A life of Hongik, of truly living for the good of all, is the best method for the growth of the soul in old age.

Alyse Gutter, who lives in New Jersey, is fully enjoying the joy of the soul through a life of Hongik. Having turned 70, she was experiencing the sadness of being parted from her husband by death two years before. She had normally thought of herself as independent and without many attachments, especially in regard to married life. But she says that she suffered greatly, physically and mentally, following her husband's death. What got her back on her feet was engaging with other people. The life lesson she learned through her experience of bereavement enabled her to understand and sympathize with the sadness and pain of others. She was able to smile again as she taught free yoga classes to the visually impaired and elderly at a community center and taught members at a yoga center. She is now aging happily and beautifully. Alyse had this to say about finding happiness:

My greatest joy is when I'm training with people. I forget my worries and forget that time is even passing; it's just joyful, beautiful, and peaceful. It's the best way for me to get up full of energy in the morning and go to sleep peacefully in the evening. A life spent sitting in a rocking chair on my porch and playing cards would be a death sentence for me now. That would be the last kind of life I would want to live. I'm not judging it in others, I'm just saying, for me, no thanks.

Ideal aging, I think, is becoming a grandmother. The grandmother I'm speaking of here means a grandmother who serves the world, people, children, and the earth. It's a life of loving each individual, a life of service for continuously sharing that love and care. People say that it's giving back, but I see it as connecting more and more, with these precious hours, precious life, the precious earth, precious people, and with my purpose, my soul. I want to complete the reason and purpose behind why I came into this world. Not just because I'm getting old, not because my hair is gradually getting whiter. I really want to live a good life for everyone and everything, a life lived caring for my body, caring for my emotions, caring for my thoughts, and sharing those methods with as many people as possible.

The Joy of Awakening

As we live our lives, we taste a profound joy when we awaken to the principles of nature and life. Especially when we enter old age, realizations happen inside us like puzzle pieces falling into place as we begin to understand, bit by bit, the essence of nature and life—once an unsolved riddle. Moment by moment, that enlightenment comes to us from the moon and stars we see in the sky, the cycle of the seasons with its budding and falling leaves, a wildflower blooming beside the road, the bright and innocent smiles of children, the wrinkles spreading across the faces of our friends. This is the joy of enlightenment. As we taste these joys in old age, we become enlightened elders.

Confucius said, "At 15, I set my heart on learning; at 30, I firmly took my stand; at 40, I had no delusions; at 50, I knew the mandate of Heaven; at 60, my ear was attuned; at 70, I followed my heart's desire without overstepping the boundaries of what was right."

Just as sharp-edged stones are ground again and again to become smooth gravel, the experiences obtained through the twists and turns of a life of 60-plus years give you a well-rounded, embracing perspective on people, life, and the world. That's why I think it is a great blessing that we have old age in life. Old age is the optimal time for awakening. It's an opportunity to make up for our shortcomings as we look back on our lives and to find closure with the wisdom we've obtained. I feel sorrow for people who meet death before they turn 60 years old. From a certain perspective, they left the world without experiencing the spiritual golden age of life, a time when we can feel the greatest spiritual abundance.

Old age is a time when we gain the ability to see the principles of all things. Perhaps this is the wisdom that time brings—not understood through facts or information, but known automatically through long experience. Those who have opened their eyes to the nature of life are enlightened elders. Just as wise elders once led the village community when it was the center of life, so, too, today's enlightened elders can become spiritual guides for the next generation through the insight and wisdom they have obtained from life and nature. The friendly, considerate advice of our grandfathers and grandmothers will resound in the hearts of the next generation, who are worrying about why they live and what they should live for.

The Joy of Creation

Those who have experienced it even once know how great the joy of creation is. For example, writers feel great delight the moment they express the messages welling up within them. They tremble with the joy of creation when they put into words the feelings that they really want to express. In that moment, it feels as if hormones of happiness and joy are being secreted in large quantities in the brain. Brain power revives at the moment of creation, and the energy of pride and satisfaction fills the heart as we think, "I expressed this!"

True satisfaction and happiness are felt when we confirm

our self-worth, when we think that we have value. People who pursue the arts—music, painting, dance, literature—have experienced this joy of creation. That's why many people start a creative hobby in their old age, such as writing, playing a musical instrument, painting, or photography. They can have their fill of the joy of creation, the joy of expressing their own inspirations.

It's not only in the arts that we can taste the joy of creation. Each and every moment we go on living our lives is an opportunity for creation. Carrying out something we feel is needed in our daily lives, improving something that feels uncomfortable, attempting something we've never tried before, taking a new approach to something—these are all acts of creation.

I believe in two immutable laws of creation.

First, there is no creation unless you act. No action, no creation. Thinking of creating something is merely the beginning. Creation doesn't happen unless you act, no matter what good thoughts you have or what good choices you make. You may have a bell right before your eyes, but unless you ring it, you won't hear its beautiful sound.

I'd like to share an experience I had. Since I was young, I've tried very hard to learn the meaning and purpose of my life. Then, at the age of 30, I realized through 21 days of extreme mind-body training that my energy was cosmic energy and that my mind was cosmic mind. The realization that my substance was one with the great life energy of the cosmos, the source of all creation, brought me great hope, joy, and peace.

After that, I started actively searching for ways to share my enlightenment. The first action I took was to get up early in the morning and go to a nearby park. I would share health practices with everyone I met. And whenever I walked down the road, if I saw someone who looked physically ill or emotionally troubled, I would feel peace only after speaking to them and giving them helpful advice. It went so far that my wife, who saw me doing this, told me that she was embarrassed to be seen with me.

I wasn't such a proactive person from the very beginning. People who see me now wouldn't believe it, but originally I was introverted, passive, and really bashful. It was through action that I was able to overcome who I was. I would waver and hesitate before taking any action, but when I actually did something, I realized it wasn't any big deal. I gradually grew more confident the more I experienced this.

In many ways, the environment I faced in the early days in 1980, when I first taught what is now known as Body & Brain Yoga, was not good. I started on the streets, in a park, without even having a decent location, but I didn't simply wait to be given a good environment. I wasn't picky about time or place. If there was someone who looked unhappy, someone who looked ill, I would go with the feeling that I should help them, no matter what. What started in that humble way is now spreading throughout South Korea, the United States, and the world, and I developed it into the academic discipline of Brain Education.

In the early days, I taught mind-body health practices for free in a park for five years because I believed my enlightenment was true. I could do that because I had the conviction that the enlightenment I had obtained was available to everyone. I kept motivating myself to move, telling myself that if enlightenment cannot be shared with others, it is not true enlightenment. No action, no creation. I was certain that the power of creation I had experienced was in everyone.

The second immutable law of creation, I believe, is that creation must begin in you. You have to be able to move your energy, your mood, in a bright, positive direction. That is the beginning of creation. You must develop in yourself a state of bright energy that permits creation. For example, if you see yourself struggling, weighed down by heavy energy as you worry and fret over things, wake up and pay attention. Get up and do one minute of exercise. Say to your body and old habits, "I am your master. I create my own life." As the energy of your body and mind changes when you do that, your brain power will revive, and your creativity will start to spark into life.

If you look around when you're in such a state, you'll find yourself surrounded by creative potential. You can bring vitality to your daily life as you smile brightly at the family members you see every day, as you share warm greetings with neighbors, or as you create meaningful time with friends. If you want to taste the joy of even greater creation, attempt something new, something you've never done before. Start a hobby you've really wanted to try, or begin doing volunteer activity for a community organization.

Instead of just vacantly watching time go by in your old age, roll up your sleeves and get involved in volunteer activity. You'll feel yourself filling with pride as you realize, "I can help other people! I can contribute something to society!"

There is nothing so fulfilling as the moments when you feel you're helping someone, for in that moment you can confirm the value of your existence. You escape from your daily tedium and change it into a succession of valuable days spent creating joy and happiness.

Are you worried that you're not happy? Then discover new sources of happiness. The joy of Hongik, the joy of awakening, and the joy of creation—these are wellsprings of new happiness that will quench your soul's thirst. And with your dedication, they will grow into a powerful waterway that leads you to the ocean of completion.

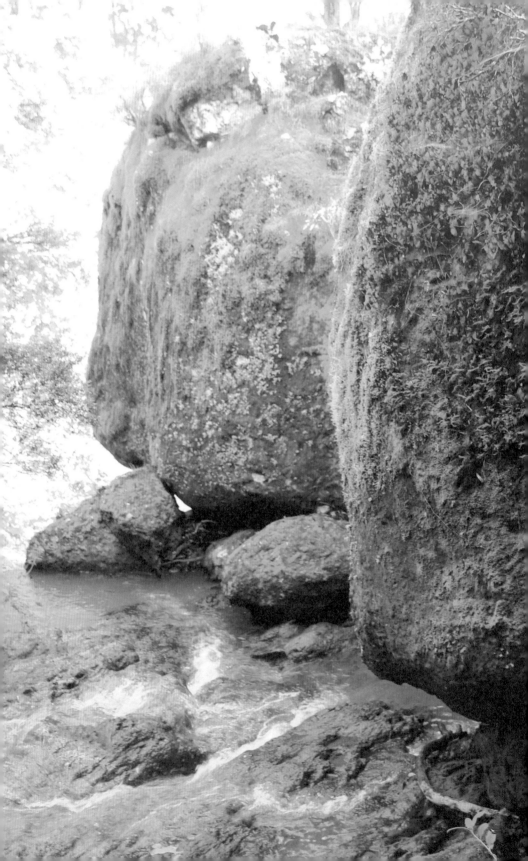

CHAPTER 7

Let Go of Attachments to Find Peace

In old age, we are able to feel peace more than at any other time in life. Once we have experienced all the tempests and emotional whirlwinds of life, most things no longer shock or overwhelm us.

Despite this, many older people—especially those who are comparatively young, in their 60s and 70s—are not free from disturbances of the mind caused by selfishness and greed. In severe cases, they are actually more narrow-minded, self-centered, and cranky than young people. Seeing such seniors, young people can't help but wrinkle their brows and think, "There's no way I'm going to grow old like that!" How many people would want to age into a selfish, greedy old person? Everyone wants to grow kinder and more peaceful as they age. What, then, can you do to become more peaceful?

As a starting point, you need to be capable of introspection, of watching yourself. You need to be able to open your mind's eye to watch your inner world. And you must check to see whether you have peace inside.

- Am I at peace now?

- Is my mind still troubled?

- If I'm not at peace, why is that?

Not being at peace means that your soul is not free, and the reason your soul is not free is that it is attached to something. Just as you can't use your hands freely if they're holding something, your soul cannot be free if your mind is clinging to something.

Things That Weigh Down Our Souls

If you can't be at peace, then clearly there's a reason for that. You are clinging to something, so your mind cannot help but be troubled. You must be able to see honestly and accurately what you're attached to. Comparing our souls to containers, the things placed in those containers are our attachments. Because of those attachments, the soul feels heavy and troubled.

The things to which people are commonly attached can be divided into three general categories.

First is attachment to wealth and material things. It would be great to have plenty of wealth and material things in old age, but it is okay just to have enough to lead your life without being needy. You no longer need to financially support parents or children, as you did when you were younger, and usually your cost of living decreases when you simplify your lifestyle. It's true that medical expenditures may increase, but you can mitigate that by consistently managing your health and physical condition. Some people need to continue earning money for quite a while into old age, but this can help them live more youthful and vigorous lives.

The problem is excessive attachment to material things. The greedy desire to earn a fortune or to enjoy wealth and luxury in old age is a poison that destroys peace of mind; living a life without great discomfort can be enough. Rather than thinking that you should earn a great deal of money by making new investments, it would be better to live a frugal life as you cut back on your spending. Furthermore, as a crowning virtue, you could share a little of what you have with those around you and use your material abundance to experience the nonmaterial joys of Hongik, awakening, and creation.

The second common attachment is to power or prestige. People want their name to be known in the world, as reflected in this Korean saying: "A tiger dies and leaves a skin; a human dies and leaves a name." We have a need for recognition; we want many people to acknowledge our existence and value. That's why, at a young age, we work constantly for success. After we're older, our attachment to power and prestige continues through various types of poor behavior.

This attachment may show itself through bragging about what you did when you were young: "Back in the day, I used to . . . ." Of course, it's perfectly fine to enjoy reminiscing about the days of your youth, when you were in the prime of your life. But continuously referring to the "good old days" suggests that you're not happy with who you are now, as though who you are now, as an older person, is not good enough. Continuously thinking and talking about the past, pining for those times, prevents you from focusing on and acting in the here and now.

Some people also remain attached to power and prestige as they get older. If you want to help make the world a better place, it is natural to want to become known for those actions, even to gain fame for them, since a good reputation can help you have greater influence on the world. If the desire for power and prestige comes first, though, the tail ends up wagging the dog, causing dissonance that ultimately boomerangs back as dishonor. Have we not witnessed many political leaders and business people being brought low by dishonor? People behave this way when the desire to gain prestige overtakes the desire to be of service to others.

To resolve your obsession with power and prestige, you have to know how to observe your need for recognition accurately. Learn to recognize yourself instead of hanging on to recognition that other people give you. The acknowledgment of our soul is greater recognition than anything else. Along with an inner feeling of pride, the greatest praise is a voice inside you saying, "Yeah, you did great!" Your soul recognizing and being satisfied with you is like Heaven recognizing you. That bright true nature, the soul within you, is Heaven.

Third, people can become attached to other people. From a certain perspective, this is the trickiest attachment to handle. Material things and power aren't living organisms, so you can let go of those attachments just by changing your mind. Unlike those inanimate objects, however, the people we meet in our personal relationships have thoughts and emotions. Our emotions are like a rugby ball; you never know where it may bounce. You may be controlling your emotions well, only to find that your composure breaks down in an instant when you're subject to an emotional attack by another person. As that happens, we hurt each other and come to dislike and resent the other person.

Attachment to somebody manifests itself in two forms: love and hate. Like two sides of a coin, these are the two forms of emotion that are always flipping back and forth in personal relationships. In fact, they have a single root: attachment.

Some people might think that because love is a good emotion, loving someone cannot be called an attachment. But the emotion of love is none other than attachment if it interferes with freeing your soul. As we live our lives, we find relationships that end in separation no matter how loving they once were, and even people who live together their whole lives must experience the unavoidable separation of death when one of them leaves the world first. How psychologically hard is it when someone you love leaves, or when you leave someone you love?

How, then, can we love without attachment? To do this, we need to maintain the freedom of our souls. You can gain the freedom of your soul when you transcend the emotion of romantic love, sublimating it as peace, a higher level of emotion. When you are centered in the freedom and peace of your soul, you will come to accept dispassionately even painful separation. Then you can have a higher level of love for others, centered not in attachment, but in the growth, freedom, and peace of each other's soul. This isn't that easy, though. Since love is an exchange between two people, it's not enough if only one person has this awareness. Both must want to be a help-mate, contributing to the growth of the other's soul.

People commonly want to possess, control, and confine other people in the name of love. That can lead to misfortune for them as well as for the other person. The emotion of love can give birth to attachment and suddenly change to hate when that attachment and greed aren't satisfied. If you continue to live without letting go of the attachment of hate, you will never be happy.

Hate occurs in ordinary personal relationships, not just loving ones. We have hate for anyone who has caused us harm, whether financial, physical, or mental. So we live without for-giving the other person, with the victim consciousness that identifies ourselves as the victim and the other as the victim-izer. If you live your whole life with victim consciousness and with hate in your heart, it cannot help but cause great pain for both you and the other person. Conversely, when you've caused great harm to someone, you end up suffering from guilt. Guilt is truly the darkest and most self-destructive form of conscious-ness, one that blocks the growth of the soul.

When we reflect on our lives in our old age, emotions such as attachment, greed, victim consciousness, and guilt may come to the forefront of our minds. We realize and regret, all too late, that these forms of consciousness made our lives dif-ficult and complicated. If we never also realize what we can do differently, we may carry this regret to the end of our days.

We have to choose for ourselves. Will we live out our lives continuously troubled by such regretful emotions, or release them and be free? It's about whether we will neglect or solve the problem. If you want a life that is truly without regret, if you want true freedom and peace of your soul, then choose the latter and actively explore solutions.

How can you resolve such negative forms of consciousness? Start by cleansing your inner self to free yourself from them.

As an example, let's look at victim consciousness, one of the most overwhelming emotions. People generally have at least one or two sources of victim consciousness. They think that they've been hurt by someone, often a person who is close, like a family member, lover, friend, or colleague, because wounds of the heart tend to be greatest in relationships that have been close.

To resolve your victim consciousness, begin by escaping from the idea that you are a victim. As long as you are immersed in that thought, you cannot cleanse the various negative emotions and forms of information that are in your subconscious mind. When you think of yourself as a victim, a victimizer appears in your subconscious mind. The more you think about the victimizer who caused you harm, the greater your hate grows. You may say to yourself, "I can never forgive the victimizer, and I curse him," or "I should make him pay because he wronged me."

Once you create one victimizer in your subconscious, the number of victimizers increases. When distrust of someone develops in your mind because of a single injury, you suspect that others, too, might harm you, and you put up your guard against them. Victim consciousness keeps creating victimizers and giving rise to negative energy. That negative energy eats away at positive energy, and in the end it weakens the body's natural healing power. It is impossible for joy, happiness, freedom, and peace of the soul to exist when negative energy is continuously expanding. There is only suffering. This is a terrifying way to immerse yourself in unhappiness.

The way to escape from victim consciousness is to quickly switch your awareness of yourself from victim to victimizer. Try to change your thinking so you realize that you're not the only one who was hurt, and that, in fact, you may have hurt the other person, too. For example, when a couple fights, it's often not the fault of only one side. If you take a closer look, you'll find that there were issues, large or small, on both sides. When you look at it only from your own perspective, it's easy to think that only you have suffered harm. But if you change your thinking to see that you were also a victimizer, you can approach the other person first and say, "I'm sorry. Please forgive me."

There will probably be times when you have truly been hurt unilaterally. What could you do in that case? Even then, change your awareness to view yourself as the victimizer. Victimizer here doesn't mean someone who has caused harm to someone else. It's a matter of taking responsibility for yourself. It's about being able to tell yourself, "I have been my own victimizer. I am the one who has made my life this way."

Why should you do that? If you are the victimizer, then changing yourself is enough to change your current situation. If you think of yourself as the victim, though, there will be limits to how much you can change unless the victimizer changes. Resentment and hatred for the perpetrator who hurt you will always be there in your conscious and subconscious mind.

Realize that you—not someone else—are the one who made you who you are and created your situation as it is now. Escape from this thought: "I'm like this because of you. It's all your fault." Think this instead: "I have chosen and created everything. I won't resent anyone. It's all my responsibility." Do that unconditionally, without making any excuses, even if it would be clear to anyone who looked at your situation that you suffered harm. You can begin anew once you have that consciousness. Your true sense of responsibility concerning your life starts to revive once you've had this change of heart. You switch to a positive mode, telling yourself, "I am the master of my life. I'll no longer resent others, wallowing in victim consciousness. Instead, I will pioneer my life." Your resentment changes to forgiveness, tolerance, and gratitude when you are the master of your life.

To have peace, you must be free from attachments. Old age is the optimal opportunity to look into the emotions you haven't been able to cleanse and to let go of your attachments, one by one. Just as a hot air balloon rises into the sky when we release the sandbags holding it down, one by one, our souls can be lighter and freer when we let go of our attachments.

Meditation for the Soul's Freedom

Let me introduce you to a method of meditation for discarding attachments and becoming a free soul.

Bring one hand in front of your chest, palm turned upward. Cup your palm as if to receive falling water. Close your eyes and imagine your hand as the cup of your soul. Once there was nothing in the cup of your soul; the weight of your soul was zero. As you've lived your life, though, you have put many different things in that cup. Those became attachments that have gradually weighed down your soul.

What does the cup of your soul hold now? What attachments are inside it? Are they attachments to wealth and material things? Attachments to power and prestige? To people you love? Is there hatred for people who have troubled you? What is it that keeps your soul from being free, that oppresses it and weighs it down? Different kinds of negative emotions and forms of consciousness? Greed, selfishness, victim consciousness, feelings of inferiority, arrogance, defeat, guilt?

Do you want to be a free soul? If you do, then let all those things go, for they are not the substance of who you are. Only one thing is your substance: your soul. Everything else is like a rock that clings to your soul. For your soul to be free, you must dump that rock, and that requires courage. Only you can make that choice. No one can force you to choose, and no one can choose for you, either.

Now count to three in your mind and slowly turn your hand over so that your palm faces down, pouring out the things contained in the cup of your soul.

One, two, three!

Completely let go of everything that burdened and troubled your soul. Feel the ardent desire to become a free soul, and feel only that desire. Feel the earnest desire in your heart to soar freely in the heavens, like a bird.

Now spread your arms to your sides and flap them up and down like the wings of a bird. Give yourself complete freedom. Slowly fly into the wide open sky.

Your energy gradually grows lighter and brighter. You are a free soul! Feel your chest opening and breathing. Fully enjoy the freedom of your soul as a smile spreads across your face.

Slowly stop moving, place your hands on your knees, and adopt a meditation posture. What are you feeling in your heart right now? Do you feel freedom and peace?

Someone whose heart is at peace is blessed. Peace of mind comes when we let go of our attachments. Attachments come from foolishness, and foolishness develops when we don't know the purpose of our lives. We become attached to money, prestige, and people when we don't know why we live, why we've come to earth, and what we should live for.

We have come to earth for the growth and completion of our souls. Though we can discard everything else, we can never discard our soul. Though we have to leave everything behind when we die, the one thing we have to take with us is our soul. Your soul is the substance and essence of who you are. For the growth and completion of your soul, you have been crying, laughing, loving, hating, and learning life's lessons in the

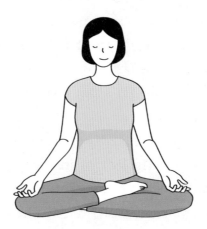

MEDITATION FOR THE SOUL'S FREEDOM

1. Bring a hand in front of your chest, palm cupped upward.

2. Close your eyes and imagine your hand as the cup of your free, pure soul.

3. See all of the attachments you have put in the cup that are weighing down your soul.

4. Turn your hand over and pour out your attachments.

5. Spread your arms to the side and flap them like the wings of a bird. Let your soul fly freely. Smile.

6. Put your hands on your knees in a meditation posture and feel your heart. Do you feel freedom and peace?

7. Place your hands on your chest, one over the other, and intend for the growth and completion of your soul. Feel the light and peace that comes to you, and have gratitude for it.

training hall of enlightenment that is life.

We have come into this life for training, for spiritual practice. Everything you have experienced, good or bad, bitter or sweet, has been meaningful and has taught you. When you realize this, gratitude and peace begin to develop in your heart. The seed of your soul starts to grow when your heart is at peace.

Place your hands on your chest, one over the other, and yearn solely for the growth and completion of your soul. Great light will come to you. The light of great wisdom teaching you where to go will shine upon you. Entrust everything to that light. Once dark, your mind and the depths of your soul will grow brighter and clearer. Your heavy chest will grow light and peaceful.

You'll feel it. "Everything happened because of my attachments! These attachments blocked my heart and troubled me!" If you've seen the eternal light and found the path of your soul, have gratitude to that bright light of wisdom that shone on you. Remember that the light of wisdom is always shining on you, and hold peace in your heart.

"

Someone whose heart is
at peace is blessed. Peace
of mind comes when we
let go of our attachments.
Attachments come from
foolishness, and
foolishness develops
when we don't know the
purpose of our lives."

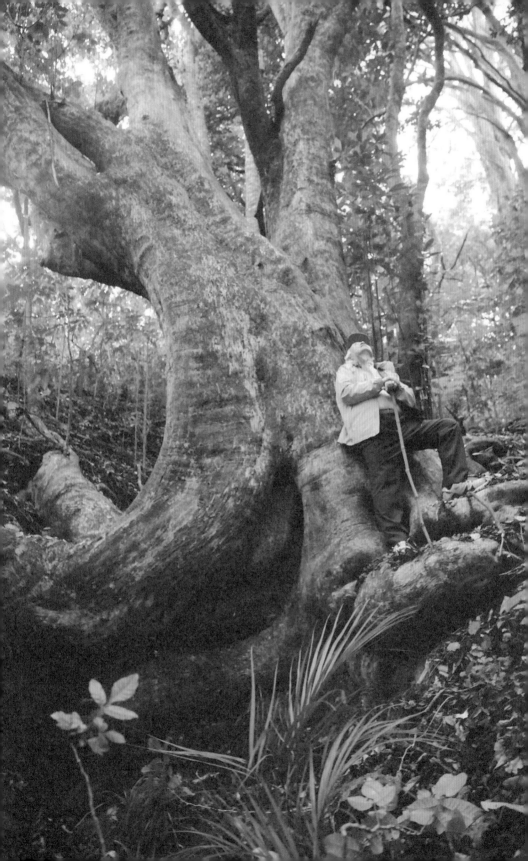

CHAPTER 8

Don't Fear
Solitude—Enjoy It

Along with economic problems and disease, one of the greatest difficulties experienced by the elderly is loneliness. Couples who once lived busy lives raising their children find themselves alone in an empty nest when those children go off to form separate families. And when an older person is separated from a spouse by death or divorce, the rest of his or her life seems inevitably lonely. According to the 2010 US census, 28 percent of people over the age of 65—10 million people—were living alone.

The isolation of the elderly doesn't only cause loneliness. It has also been shown to have a negative impact on physical and mental health, increasing conditions like chronic disease, high blood pressure, depression, cognitive decline, and dementia. Conversely, people who are connected with family and friends and have meaningful personal relationships are not only physically and mentally healthier, they also have longer life expectancies. Having people around us with whom we can communicate on a heart-to-heart level may also reduce the effects of stress. It's not enough to communicate by text or email, says psychologist Susan Pinker. "Face-to-face contact releases a whole cascade of neurotransmitters and, like a vaccine, they protect you now in the present and well into the future."

Humans are social animals. We have to live with and among other people if our happiness is to increase and we are to get a real taste of life. But the loneliness I want to speak about in this chapter is a little different from the loneliness we experience when we lack enough meaningful relationships. It is the fundamental solitude of being that comes in old age. Even if someone we love is right next to us, this solitude is of a different depth from the passing loneliness we may experience in our youth. Moments of sudden realization concerning our existence—standing between life and death—may come as we see friends departing for the next world, one by one. Death, which once seemed far off, gradually approaches as a reality that we will have to face directly. And the realization that we will have to depart alone on the path of death, that it is a solitary path we must travel with no one to accompany us, grows deeper little by little. When the essential aloneness of being, a loneliness that we cannot find any way to relieve, comes rushing over us, how can we deal with it?

Learning How to Enjoy Solitude

I want to say this to you: Don't fear loneliness; accept it. And enjoy solitude.

Everyone comes into the world alone and leaves it alone. So a human is originally a lonely being. Young or old, rich or poor, famous or unknown, a president or a street cleaner, every-one experiences moments when the loneliness of existence suddenly touches them deep within.

Some seek other people to alleviate that loneliness, while some are addicted to alcohol, drugs, sex, or various forms of entertainment. Some live mired in depression or give up in despair because they can't endure the loneliness. Others, though, face the substance of their loneliness head on and experience an awakening of consciousness through deep reflection on the essence of human life. They choose life on a new level of spiritual maturity, and they gain inner joy from the experience. I don't believe that such a life is limited to special people who pursue spirituality. We are all born with a spiritual nature. What's important is how we sublimate loneliness regarding the essence of our being.

Life is a long journey meant for leaping beyond loneliness to find unchanging freedom and truth. This is humanity's craving for enlightenment, and through that enlightenment, loneliness is no longer dark and depressing but changes into *brilliant solitude*. Unenlightened loneliness is dark and trying. Brilliant solitude, though, shines brightly, and that light shines on those around us. The moon in the sky is alone, but its light shines brightly in the darkness. In the same way, brilliant light shines from those who have gained insight into the true meaning of life by facing solitude with courage.

Old age is the optimal time for gaining such insight, I believe. While physical eyes look at the world and people in reality, each of us can be an enlightened elder whose mind's eye is always open to nature and the universe. Let's not avoid being solitary in old age. Continue learning how to make friends with solitude, how to enjoy solitude. Just as Confucius said that he understood the mandate of Heaven at the age of 50, so we, too, should go forward with our eyes lifted to Heaven in our old age. We should be enlightened elders, our heads raised toward Heaven, embracing people and the world and walking toward completion.

The Fragrance of Brilliant Solitude

I established my own purpose at the age of 30 and started sharing it with people in a small park. When you have a purpose and a vision in your heart, there are times you are destined to go against the current instead of just flowing with it. There will be adversities, obstacles, and misunderstandings in the course of opening up a path not traveled by others. There have been times when I was lonely, times when I was afraid, times when I was sad, and many times when I felt that I was standing completely alone on a barren plain. At such times, I would look up into the night sky. I felt that I could open my heart only to the stars in the sky. There are countless stars in the dark night sky, but each one seemed lonely, like me. Yet those stars were shining, even in that loneliness.

That was brilliant solitude, a time for completely returning to the source of my existence. That solitude was a time of enlightenment and creation. I encountered who I really was in that solitude. I felt that the only stars able to illuminate me were my conviction and my vision. I wasn't able to let go of that vision because, if I did, there would only be eternal darkness around me. So I made this pledge:

> Now that I have found a dream and am traveling my own path, the sadness that comes from failing to get the understanding of others is nothing. But giving up my dream is death for me. I will walk this path even if no one in the world can understand me. I will remain true to this dream though everyone in the world abandons it.

In solitude, my conviction has continued to grow stronger and stronger.

The soul headed toward completion feels brilliant solitude. You enjoy this solitude as you live within it. It's not a solitude you share with others; it's a fullness that comes in the moment when, alone, you connect with everything as one. When you look at the stars in the night sky, when you walk on a quiet path through the woods, when you watch the setting sun, when you meditate and practice alone—these moments come to you when you're alone yet connected with all things. These are the moments when you taste brilliant solitude. This is when you realize that the fundamental loneliness within you can never be filled by another person or by anything outside you, that this lonely emptiness is only filled by being completely one with the great life force of the universe.

The solitude of those who have firm convictions and a vision to support their lives is like the backbone in our body. Try straightening your lower back completely. Your spine supports heaven above and connects to the earth below. Your whole body will feel comfortable only if your spine is centered exactly. Your body will feel uncomfortable if your spine leans toward your left shoulder, toward your right hip, toward your front or your back. Each part of your body, including your internal organs, is more comfortable when your spine is correctly aligned. Those who would complete their souls in brilliant solitude must think of their upright spines. With their heads lifted toward heaven and their feet firmly on the ground, they must live lives of embracing the brilliant solitude in their hearts and sharing pure love, the energy of their souls, with others.

Do not fear loneliness. Great wisdom and love come to us from solitude and loneliness. The path of a human is essentially lonely, but when that solitude has reached the extreme and gone beyond, it changes to great gladness and peace. That's when you know great compassion. Great compassion can be felt when it transcends human affection. It's easy for human affection to give birth to attachment. When you are leaning to one side and relying on or stuck in something, you cannot feel the whole. You feel the whole when you are completely alone and lonely. When the loneliness of being reaches deep into your heart, a bright light breaks out of the darkness. Then great solitude changes into brilliant light.

If you go forward with brilliant solitude in your heart, you become what I call a truly fragrant person, one who has the greatest possible attractiveness, like a flower that must be admired for its beauty. Then you develop a character that stands firmly in its center without attaching itself to other people or running from them or pushing them away. You become able to find the seat of harmony—an encompassing public peace and public love. You are able to feel the greatest world of consciousness that can be felt by a human being. The wisdom and power to bring harmony to the world emerges when you can look at the world with this awareness.

Unenlightened loneliness is dark
and trying. Brilliant solitude,
though, shines brightly, and that
light shines on those around us."

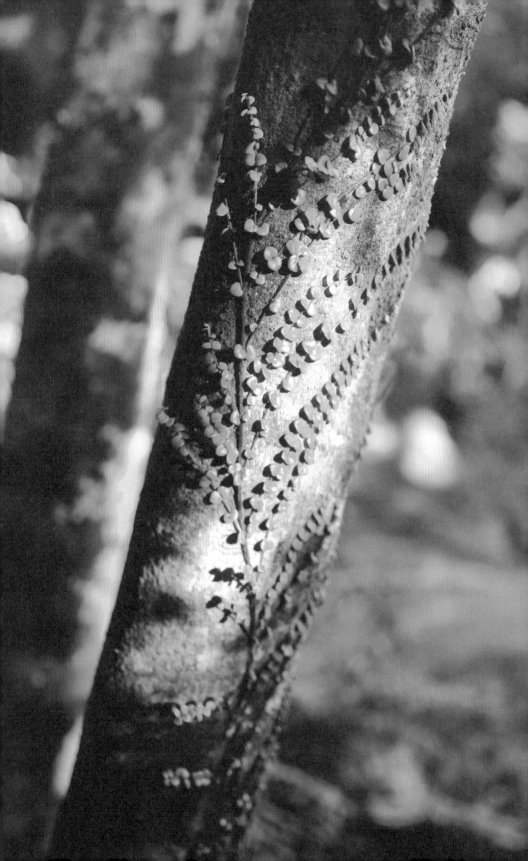

CHAPTER 9

Give Your Brain
Hopes and Dreams

When they get together, older people often joke about those senior moments that really make them feel their age. They tell stories about how somebody went from his living room into his bedroom but couldn't remember why, how he rummaged through the whole room searching for glasses that he was wearing, how he was embarrassed when he couldn't remember the name of someone he meets often, or how he parked his car in the garage but forgot to turn off the engine. Such stories often lead to worry: "I'm so forgetful. Am I going to end up suffering from dementia?"

Are hurting all over and worsening memory unavoidable physiological symptoms that we all experience as we get older? Brain scientists say no. The things we accept as a natural part of aging are, in fact, mostly the result of bad habits and healthcare, they say, not simply being old. For example, dementia doesn't develop because you are 60 or 70 years old; it appears as a symptom that results from bad eating and lifestyle habits, lack of exercise, brain injury, and so on—things that have accumulated over decades. Yes, a family history can make some types of dementia, but for the most part, we can protect the health of our brain just as we do the rest of our body.

Some people suffer from physical weakness and chronic illness even in their 20s, while others overflow with vitality in their 80s. Some still look at the world with young, curious eyes and are interested in everything around them in old age, but many shut the doors of their minds against new things even at a young age. Scientific research shows that body and brain health do not deteriorate naturally with age. Rather, the rate of aging differs significantly from person to person, depending on how well we take care of ourselves.

Only a few decades ago, brain scientists thought that our brain structure was completed sometime after the age of 20 and changed almost not at all after that. The commonly accepted theory was that neurons die continuously after birth, their numbers decreasing and no new cells developing. Now, however, we know that our brains constantly change from the moment we are born until the time we die. Not only do new neurons develop even when we're older, but new networks are created between neurons, and brain function can improve.

Of course, certain phenomena of aging do take place in our brains as we get older, just as they occur in our bodies. In the same way that our muscles grow weaker if we don't use them, parts of our brains that we don't use become less effective. Memory, concentration, and reaction time decrease in old age unless we train the brain's cognitive functions. We can keep our brains young and healthy, though, if we take good care of them and train them well. Our brains have incredible resilience. This is a great hope for all of us, for no matter how old we are, we can learn and experience new things and change our thoughts and habits. It's easy to think that people don't change much and that it's especially hard to change when we get older. But people *can* change. In fact, they are changing every moment, no matter how old they are, thanks to the brain's amazing plasticity. It's important that we guide the direction of that change by training our brains.

More than 20 years ago, I put together principles and methods for developing and using the brain's potential, creating a system of self-development that I called Brain Education. When I first told people about Brain Education, the public perception of the brain was quite different from what it is now. Back then, it was rare for anyone other than doctors and researchers to talk about the brain in everyday conversation. When I told people they could take care of their brain health themselves instead of entrusting it entirely to experts, some were afraid, as if I had mistakenly touched a hazardous object that shouldn't be messed with.

Now the idea that we can manage our own brain health just as we manage our physical health is widespread. This change is extremely fortunate, since we can't do anything without using our brains. In addition to the thinking and memory roles we commonly attribute to the brain, basic physiological functions for maintaining life, such as blood pressure, heart rate, body temperature, and hormones, are controlled by the brain. To manage your brain is to manage your life. When your brain improves, everything in your life improves.

Fortunately, anyone can understand the set of skills

needed to manage the brain. The earlier you learn these skills, the better, and then you will need to improve and refine them throughout your life. Old age is no exception. This is a time when it's easy for the brain to get rusty unless it's managed well, so you must manage your brain more actively now than at any other time in your life.

Give Your Brain Vitamin H

The basic needs of life are the same in our later years as they are at any age, and everything that makes a healthy person makes a healthy brain. So, if you want to make your brain healthy, develop good lifestyle habits that contribute to the health of your mind and body—get plenty of sleep, exercise regularly, eat balanced meals, and engage in appropriate social activities.

There is one thing, though, that stands above the rest as necessary nutrition for the human body, mind, and spirit: hope. Without hope, there is no drive even to live, and the more hope we have, the more motivated and enthusiastic we feel. Hope is the most powerful supplement available to us, and thankfully, we can make hope for ourselves any time just by changing our thoughts and attitudes. Whether you're eight or 80, hopes and dreams are the best way to activate and engage your brain.

A study led by Patrick Hill of Carleton University in Ottawa, Canada followed more than 6,000 participants for 14 years. People who had a goal in life were found to have a risk of death 15 percent lower than those who did not. Finding a goal helps you live longer regardless of when you find that purpose, the study showed, but the earlier someone comes to a direction for life, the earlier the positive effects are evident. Greater purpose in life consistently predicted lower mortality risk across the lifespan, showing the same benefit for younger, middle-aged, and older participants during the follow-up period, Hill said. He added, "There are a lot of reasons to believe that being purposeful might help protect older adults more so than younger ones." The results of this research were published in a 2014 edition of *Psychological Science*.

Purposeful people also have a lower probability of suffering from dementia, according to study results published by Patricia Boyle, PhD, in the *Archives of General Psychiatry* in 2012.

I can speak with greater confidence because of these research results, but in fact, this principle is obvious when you think about it. People who have purpose, who have hopes and dreams, will naturally be more positive about their lives and more proactive in their self-care—exercising more, eating better, and managing their stress. These attitudes toward life produce results that accumulate over time, naturally contributing to long-term brain health and longevity.

You could say that I developed Brain Education for this purpose: to give hope. In this system, there are five key steps— Brain Sensitizing, Brain Versatilizing, Brain Refreshing, Brain Integrating, and Brain Mastering—and dozens of training methods for each step. The first three steps are a process for relaxing body and mind and for reflecting on and releasing the emotions, thought patterns, and beliefs that act negatively on your efforts to create your destiny positively. The next two steps are a process for discovering who you are and what you want, and for redesigning your life based on this. All the steps are very simple, and all are moving you toward fully recovering hope for yourself and the world.

While the needs of human beings may change over the course of a lifetime, I believe the need for hope always predominates, regardless of age. With Brain Education, we've been especially successful in reaching out to children who are in socioeconomic conditions that have left them without any hope for their future, and research has confirmed its benefits.

A good example is the El Salvador Brain Education Project, which was started in 2011 by the IBREA FOUNDATION. This is an NGO I founded in 2008, which has Consultative Status with the United Nations Economic and Social Council. After a pilot project of just three months of daily Brain Education classes by IBREA FOUNDATION, students at a school in one of the most violent areas of El Salvador showed statistically significant improvement in test anxiety, trauma symptoms, self-regulation, and peer relationships. As the successful project expanded to four schools and then nationwide, more positive effects could be seen in the students and overall school culture. Children recovered their laughter and started to feel hope.

Gloria Mueller is the principal of Joaquin Rodezno School, one of the schools in El Salvador's capital city of San Salvador, where the program was implemented. When I met her a few years ago, the story she shared with me was striking:

Our school is in one of the most violent areas of my city. Students were immersed in drugs, and over half the students in a grade were involved in gangs. Disheartened by students high on drugs, teachers were afraid of them and all they did was try not to offend them.

After we incorporated Brain Education into our curriculum, things started to be different. The first change was significant improvement in students' academic performance. Violence and drug use also noticeably decreased. But what struck me most were the positive changes in their self-regulation and relationships.

A cocaine addict, 17-year-old Jose (not his real name) had been thrown out of his home. He had been coming to school only to get drugs. After taking the Brain Education pilot program, he was able to overcome his drug habit and is now preparing to transition to a higher grade.

Teachers witnessed how children who once didn't have any expectations about the future began to talk about their goals and dreams. Now I can see that teachers' motivation has dramatically improved.

Following a series of successful cases, 10 percent of El Salvador's public schools are currently implementing Brain Education through IBREA FOUNDATION's project in the country. The El Salvador Ministry of Education fully supports the program and has seen how it is creating sustainable results inside the schools. Besides El Salvador, Brain Education has brought hope to students and communities in the United States, South Korea, Japan, Africa, and Europe. Young students of Brain Education, especially those in relatively poor and challenging environments, taught me the importance of the power to choose hope. When they experienced love and respect for themselves, they started to look to the future with confidence rather than despair.

I believe that seniors today are not really all that different than these children. Like them, many seniors feel like they've been tossed aside, as though society as a whole has little value for them. And since we're living longer, many of us are living decades of our lives in this condition. This is a true human tragedy; just as too many kids are starting their lives without hope, too many seniors are ending their lives without hope. It has been such a joy to see Brain Education practitioners who have reached the second half of their lives rediscover their hope and enjoy vibrant lives.

Hope, after all, is a perfect source of power. Why? You can create something new if you have hope, even in a situation where you have nothing else, and you can overcome difficulties in any desperate situation if you have hope. No preconditions are required for choosing hope. You don't have to be young, have a lot of money, or have any special talent. Hope is something you just find. You discover hope for yourself—and if you can't find it, then you create it.

When we choose hope, our brains secrete large quantities of positive hormones and move our hearts with new expectations, warming them with joy and passion. A brain without hope is like a gas station that has run out of fuel. If we abandon hope, worry and fear take its place. Without hope, your brain grows weaker, no matter how much good food you eat, how diligently you exercise, or how many crossword puzzles you solve. Brains live on dreams. And brains are as active as their dreams allow, no more. The secret to living with vitality in your old age—maintaining a youthful, healthy brain—is to inspire your brain with hopes and dreams.

Remind your brain of this wonderful prose poem by Samuel Ullman, popularized by US General Douglas MacArthur:

Nobody grows old by merely living a number of years.
People grow old by deserting their ideals.
Years may wrinkle the skin, but to give up enthusiasm
*   wrinkles the soul.*
Worry, doubt, self-distrust, fear, and despair—
these are the long, long years
that bow the head and turn
the growing spirit back to dust.

You may think, "I'm retired now, so the important work of my life is over. I no longer have anything to look forward to and no hope, either." The moment you think this way, your brain switches to low energy mode. Your energy declines even though you eat the same three meals a day as you did before. Your body is limp like a soggy piece of cotton, and you find that you don't have much ambition to meet new people or try new activities.

Secretion of serotonin and dopamine, which let us feel joy and happiness, decreases.

When you lose hope, your brain chooses the status quo over new challenges. Even if opportunities come your way, it backs away from them, saying, "At my age? You must be kidding." When you give up the thought of creating a tomorrow that is better than today, your brain ages and becomes helpless. It starts emitting that energy of helplessness to your whole body and to the world around you.

"I'm retired now, so I guess I'll just take care of my grand-kids, or whatever." Friends who are in the habit of saying things like this age rapidly. Their lives are so monotonous that even their conversations are boring, including little that is new. Conversely, friends who have hopes and dreams even after retiring find things they want to do, living vigorously while engaging in passionate activities. When you meet those friends, conversations are joyful, and you can give each other positive stimuli and inspiration.

If You Think You're Old, You'll Get Old

The kind of information you give your brain is important. If you keep dreaming, actively designing the rest of your life, your brain will be filled with hope and a new sense of expec-tation. It will help you keep your body and mind health-ier, fully mobilizing your muscles, bones, organs, nervous system, and hormones.

Many studies show that thinking positively or negatively about aging actually affects your quality of life in old age, as well as your lifespan. According to one study led by Professor Andrew Steptoe of University College London, people who thought of themselves as younger than their actual age lived approximately 50 percent more years during the course of the study than those who thought of themselves as older than they are.

Even more surprising, some research has shown that when we think, "I'm old," our brain's abilities decline. Dr. Thomas Hess of North Carolina State University performed memory tests on people ages 60 through 82 and compared those who thought negatively about their age and memory with those who had a positive outlook. Individuals who had negative attitudes about their age scored lower. In other words, negative thoughts such as "My memory is poor because I'm old" or "My memory is going to be poor because I'm an old man, and people despise me because of this" actually make memory worse.

According to a 2016 report on a two-year study of 4,135 older people in Ireland, participants who had negative attitudes toward aging walked more slowly and had worse cognitive abilities than those who had a more positive outlook. Interestingly, exactly the same results were seen even when changes in medications or other factors affecting mood and health were taken into consideration. Deidre Robertson, PhD, lead researcher for the study, said, "The way we think, speak, and write about aging directly affects our health. Everyone ages, but if we have a negative attitude toward aging throughout our lives, it can have a measurable, harmful effect on our mental, physical, and cognitive health."

You've probably heard about the placebo and nocebo effects. The placebo effect is a phenomenon by which even a fake medicine with no efficacy at all has a real effect if the user believes it will be effective. In contrast, the nocebo effect is when a medication that is actually effective is shown to have no effect in users who don't believe in its potency. Both show us the powerful impact that our thoughts can have on our bodies and minds.

Giving ourselves positive, hopeful messages in our old age is critical for brain health. The brain operates most vigorously and exhibits its highest performance when we are joyful, when we feel happy, and when we think of ourselves as noble beings.

Information is brain food. Just as we need to concern ourselves with the food we eat to protect our physical health, we need to concern ourselves with information for the sake of our brain's health. If you eat the wrong food, you may get indigestion or food poisoning, gain or lose weight, become sick, or even die. In the same way, some information gives us hopes and dreams, while other information makes us discouraged, angry, or sad. Good information makes a good brain, just as healthy food makes a healthy body.

What sort of messages and information are you giving your brain concerning old age? What information are you accepting from others? Boldly reject socially accepted ideas that don't help you live your later years in health, happiness, and fullness. No matter how much depressing information the media pumps out, you can decide what attitude you will have about growing old. The second half of life is a time when we can complete our lives as we desire. Love this time and consider it precious and meaningful. Ceaselessly inspire your brain with messages that bring you expectation, passion, dreams, and hopes.

Don't Leave Your Brain in Its Default Mode

Lisa Feldman Barrett, professor of psychology at Northeastern University in Boston, Massachusetts, recently wrote a fascinating article for *The New York Times* about a study of superagers. Superagers are people whose biological age is more than 80 but who are no different from 25-year-olds in brain functions such as memory and concentration.

What areas of the brains of superagers are activated more than those of ordinary seniors? Study findings indicate that the areas that handle emotion or sentiment, not those involved with cognition or thinking, are the ones that are most activated, contradicting what common sense would have us expect. What can we do, then, to keep these areas of the brain as active as when we were young? "Keep doing difficult tasks, whether mental or physical," Professor Barrett suggests.

A high level of activity in these areas of the brain causes us to feel negative emotions such as tiredness and frustration. These are the feelings we get when we wrestle with a difficult math problem or push ourselves to our physical limits during exercise. You may develop uncomfortable weariness of body and mind when you have to focus intensely mentally, but you can develop your mental muscles to give yourself a sharper memory and more powerful focus.

I'm glad whenever I come across such articles, because it seems that the convictions I've developed through my own experiences are being supported by scientific research. Living a comfortable, easy, worry-free life isn't what's best for brain health. For the health of your brain, you need to raise its workload. It's important not to leave your brain in its default state, doing what it's always done, but instead constantly give it new tasks and stimulation.

Usually, once they're old, people don't stimulate their brains much. From the brain's perspective, it's as if its boss doesn't inspire it to work hard. A basic principle of the brain's operation is that it improves when stimulated and declines without stimulation. Hopes and dreams are the greatest stimuli we can give our brains. Our brains are highly active when our lives have purpose, direction, and plans.

Seniors can no longer use age as an excuse, claiming that a rusty brain keeps them from doing or learning something new. Our brains are able to learn until the final moments of our lives. However, learning doesn't happen smoothly without repetition and practice, no matter how flexible or good at learning our brains may be. We must have the will to keep experiencing and learning new things, and we must work through the irritating repetition and difficulties we face in the process of learning. And we need to remember that the decades we're given after we retire provide us with plenty of time to achieve something through constant repetition and training, even things we have never done before.

Brain Meditation for Positive Energy

Consciously repeating thoughts to yourself that will have a positive impact on your future is commonly called positive affirmation. I call it giving your brain positive messages and information.

To properly convey messages to your brain, you must first be clear about what you want. If you don't really know what you want in your life, you won't be able to communicate it strongly to your brain. Try taking some time to check what is important and meaningful to you as you answer the questions presented in Chapter 4 of this book. Once you are clear about what you really want, express it in writing on a piece of paper. As an example, this is a message I often give my brain these days:

> I'm overflowing with a life force that will allow me to live to 120. I'm filled with the energy of infinite love and creation. I will complete the Earth Village as I live to 120 in health and happiness.

Write down your own message, one you want to give to your brain. Make it short, positive, and written in the first person— an "I" message. This doesn't have to be a fixed message; you can change it whenever you want, and it will change naturally as you grow.

Even if you give your brain good messages, it won't be able to accept them easily when your body is tense and your mind is a tangle of thoughts, just as you have a hard time hearing someone talk when you're in a noisy place. To enable your brain to accept the messages you give it, you have to quiet your body and mind through relaxation. The following training method lets you do this quickly and easily.

Sit comfortably in a chair or on the floor. Lift your hands and tap your head with the tips of your relaxed fingers. Gently tap your whole head for two to three minutes—the top of your head, your forehead, the sides and back of your head, and the place where your neck and head meet. Relax your facial muscles and jaw, and open your mouth slightly. By tapping your head to stimulate its important energy points, you can release stagnant energy and cause fresh energy to circulate. As the once-blocked energy is released, you'll find yourself exhaling slowly with your mouth, "Hooo . . . ." After you finish tapping, sweep your head and face several times with the palms of your hands.

Now make loose fists with your hands. Alternating hands, gently tap your lower abdomen, using the lower part of your fists (where your little fingers are). The exact spot to tap is your lower dahnjon, two inches below your navel. Tapping there— the body's main energy center—strengthens the body's energy and causes it to heat up.

When your motions have developed a rhythm, start shaking your head gently from side to side. The point isn't to think about anything; just shake your head as if you were shaking out all your thoughts. Discharge your heavy, stagnant energy by continuing to breathe out through your mouth. You will feel your breathing becoming lighter and more natural as blockages in your chest open up and your tension is released. This creates an energetic state—head cool, chest open, abdomen warm—that allows your body and brain to function optimally. Continue for three to five minutes and then stop. With your eyes closed, quietly try to get a sense of your breathing as you inhale and exhale slowly about five times.

I call this Brain Wave Vibration. You can watch a video that teaches you this brain training method at Live120YearsBook.com. Another approach that can have a similar effect is Belly Button Healing, introduced in Chapter 5 of this book.

Your brain is now ready to accept messages. Quietly close your eyes and tell your brain the message you've written down. For example, if you want to give it the message "I'm filled with the energy of infinite love and creation," then visualize it is already accomplished. Imagine the energy of infinite love and creation within you, experiencing it as an energy phenomenon. Keep picturing and imagining that energy filling you. The energy system of our bodies and the operation of our brains are amazing in their greatness and perfection. Imagine a lemon right now, and your mouth will fill with saliva; you immediately feel what you've imagined. It's the law of energy: the mind creates energy. If you continue to visualize what you want, you will be able to attract such energy.

Now keep repeating, out loud or to yourself, a phrase that you want to say to your brain. You could even record and play back the message in your own voice, whatever makes you feel it as vividly as possible. Do this with a sincere, earnest heart, and you will be able to attract and manifest energy that is as powerful as you are sincere and earnest. Then, at some moment, you will feel your message moving you deeply, giving you strength and will.

When you finish this meditation, express your gratitude to your brain and your soul. Say you are thankful that they have done their best to support you and that you will make good use of the infinite creativity in your brain and the great love of the soul in your heart until the last moment of your life. Do so with all your heart.

Our Brains Lead Us to Completion

When we get older and have experienced life's many ups and downs, we come to the wisdom to awaken ourselves to the truths of life and principles of nature. Studies show that in old age we make wiser decisions because we control our emotions better and are less impulsive. Changes in our brains make us less reliant on dopamine, the hormone that makes us feel good.

When we enter old age, we have time for reflection and contemplation. As the finiteness of our lives hits home, we reflect on how we have lived so far and think seriously about what we will leave behind. We also think about what it is that brings us true happiness and meaning, since we have learned from experience that material success and possession are not all there is to life. In that sense, our spiritual sensitivity matures more in old age than at any other stage of life.

Meditating while focusing quietly on your breath, looking at new leaves sprouting on a tree to greet the spring, welcoming with a big hug a grandson who is rushing to meet you, saying goodbye to a departed loved one and remembering the traces he or she left in your life—at such moments, have you ever had the feeling that life isn't something finite that appears with your birth and disappears with your death, that it existed before you and will exist after you disappear? This is the feeling that you're connected with that infinite, eternal something, transcending space and time. It's the feeling of not lacking anything, of just being filled with infinite gratitude and peace.

These spiritual experiences are phenomena arising in our brains. Our brains are organs with unimaginable functions and potential, the most complex and sophisticated devices in the world. I am fascinated by the human brain, which causes us to question what we are, enables us to transcend the small self and expand our consciousness to the big self in our search for answers, and empowers us to discover the divine nature hidden in each moment of our ordinary lives. I'm grateful that we humans have been given such brains. I am awestruck by the care of the Creator, who designed us so that the spiritual senses of our brains would mature in our period of completion more than at any other time.

Asking ourselves who we really are, searching for an answer to that question, and becoming our true selves—this is really our greatest task in life and the greatest motivation we can give our brains. A life of completion through which we can fully realize our absolute value is the greatest dream and hope we can have in our old age. Our brains are prepared to perfectly support our journey toward completion. Anyone can experience completion as long as they maintain the will and passion to head toward that goal, and the humility and gratitude to learn and grow through experience.

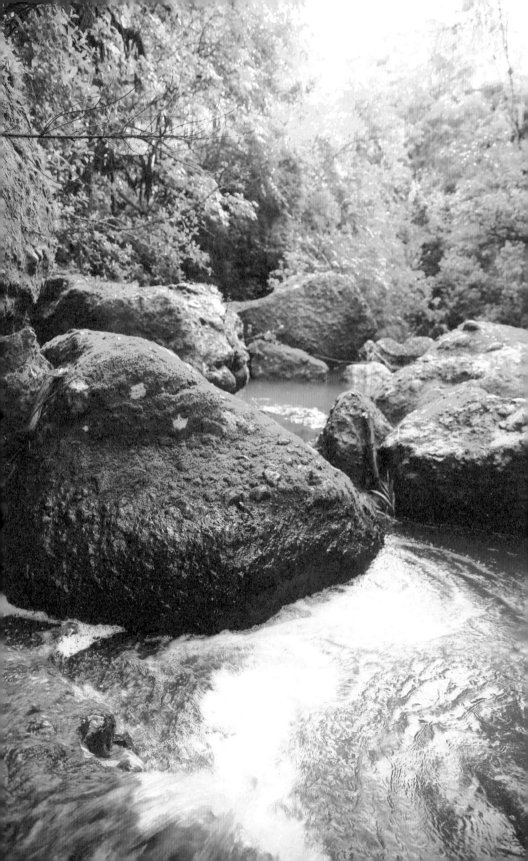

CHAPTER 10

Cultivate Yourself Continuously

Once you have lived the first half of your life, how many things will have happened to you? How many desires and emotional ups and downs will you have experienced? In the process of riding the waves of desires and emotions, pleasant and unpleasant, you'll have studied what life is automatically; you wouldn't have been able to avoid it, even if you had tried. That's why I consider old age the optimal time for awakening. Now more than ever before, you have plenty of time, and conditions are right for becoming free from responsibilities toward your family and society and for fully focusing on yourself. The life experiences and skills you've acquired provide a rich environment for the study of the mind.

Three Realizations about Life

In my book *Living Tao: Timeless Principles for Everyday Enlightenment*, I introduced three realizations concerning life. If you're a senior, by now you definitely will have come to understand at least two of these three, thanks to your lifelong experiences.

Life is suffering. This is the first realization. Anyone who has lived for 60 years will have keenly felt that life truly is suffering. Although we don't know why, we awake to find that we have been born into this world, and since we have bodies, we have to go on living. Every day, we have to feed our bodies, wash them, clothe them, put them to sleep. We have to rush around to satisfy all their needs and the desires that come from them. As we grow older, we gradually realize that all those ups and downs of life are a kind of suffering that we wouldn't have had to endure had we not been born into this world. That's why in Buddhism it is said that life itself is suffering.

Life is transient. The elderly learn this next stage of realization through direct experience. People in their 60s and 70s may be at a relatively early age for feeling that life is ephemeral. When they enter their 80s, though, and death grows closer, they cannot avoid the feeling that life seems to have little purpose. Why? Because sooner or later we have to leave everything behind. We cannot take with us the wealth we've acquired in this world, the wonderful clothes and accessories, or even a single strand from the hair on our heads. We have to leave, letting everything material and physical fall away. When death approaches, we may feel that life is really pointless. "I lived my whole life struggling so much, but I can't take anything with me! I have to leave it all behind! For what, for whom, did I struggle so much?" Thinking such things, we may find ourselves immersed in regret over the lives we've lived.

If you're a senior who has experienced these two realizations, you've attained a considerable level in the study of the mind. The problem is that while many people understand that life is suffering and transient, they fail to go on to the next level. Many passively let the years go by without any hopes or dreams, immersed in feelings of futility over life's impermanence. "What could I do at this age? It's best to just live comfortably and die quietly," they think, living the same way day in and day out, meaninglessly going through the motions, back and forth like the pendulum on a clock.

Think carefully about it, though. If you felt that life was ephemeral and stopped there, if that was the end of it, could there be a more meaningless life than that? Have we come into the world and struggled so much for nothing more than to feel that sense of futility? Do you want that to be the last spiritual insight you gain in this world? Probably not. If there really is meaning to life, then clearly there must be a stage of realization that comes after conquering nihilism. And everyone born into this world should leave it having gained that realization, for only then will life finally have meaning.

The third realization of life, what is it? When we say that life is suffering and futile, the life we speak of is a life centered on the body—in other words, on the ego. If you have seen through the illusions to grasp this all-too-obvious fact and understand the limits of life centered on the body, then you may have a feel for the nature of the life that exists beyond it. That's right: the soul, the unseen spiritual world. The soul is our substance and the essence of life.

The soul is not the ego. The soul feels shackled when the ego is present. In that state, the soul cannot be free, cannot be at peace, and cannot grow. In my earlier description of the completion of the soul, I said that in the process of Chunhwa, the energy of the soul in the heart grows and rises to the brain, where it must unite with the energy of divinity. When our souls encounter and unite with the divine nature, we experience incredible joy and peace along with a great, bright light. That is the third realization, the concept of *nothingness*, or *mu* in Korean.

The literal meaning of the word mu is not to exist, but it is a concept that transcends existence and nonexistence. It is a state of cosmic unity in which you transcend your small self, your ego, to become one with the universe. Nothingness is not a material concept; it signifies the great life energy of the cosmos. It is the infinite source of life, the world of energy, which is made up of being and nonbeing, the visible and invisible, matter and spirit. This, then, is the third realization: *The body and ego are not my essence; the great life energy of the cosmos is the substance of who I am, and I am one with all things.* This is called *muah* in Korean (literally "no-self"), meaning a state in which I have awakened to my big self, which is one with the universe, not my small self, my ego.

Do you want to end your life after living halfheartedly in the awareness that life is suffering and meaningless? Or do you want to end your life realizing that your substance is one with the infinite life energy of the cosmos and living for peace and completion, for Chunhwa? I believe that all seniors can grasp this third realization, and I hope that they will. Only when we have felt this can our lives finally escape from suffering and anguish. For then we have realized the way of Chunhwa, which says that we are one with the great life energy of the cosmos and that the place we will return after we die is also the source of that life energy.

But just because you've realized this doesn't mean that you're finished. Enlightenment is just the beginning, not the end. What's important is living an awakened life, a spiritual life. If you're curious about what a spiritual life is, then think about the opposite, about what a physical life is. A physical life is centered around the needs of the body. Compared with that, a spiritual life is centered around the growth and completion of the soul.

We have a lot of life left even after feeling the third realization. What should you do during that time? An ideal spiritual life during old age means developing that realization as you put it into practice. A life centered on the growth of the soul, not the needs of the ego, begins now in earnest. This is the second half of your life, a life lived for completion after the age of 60.

I propose three concrete elements for living a spiritual life. The first is sustained self-cultivation, the second is Hongik— the sharing and giving of benevolence, and the third is being close to nature. A combination of these three elements is perfect for the completion of the soul. In this chapter, I will talk about self-development, and in the following chapters I will deal with a life of Hongik and getting close to nature.

Continuously Train Your Body, Mind, and Spirit

At the heart of self-cultivation lies continuous training of body, mind, and spirit. Physical exercise, like the One-Minute Exercise program I talked about in Chapter 5, is a good way to train mind and spirit as well as body. Never stop exercising as long as you have strength left to move your body, like 105-year-old cyclist Robert Marchand, who exercises an hour a day. That is the most fundamental of fundamentals.

But there is something I highly recommend in addition to physical exercise: meditation.

The essence of meditation is to be fully in the moment. Generally, our minds are full of complex thoughts, positive or negative. Instead of being in the here and now, our minds wander all over the place, chasing after thoughts, feelings, or the sensual stimuli or information surrounding us. Meditation is about bringing your mind back to the here and now, observing and recognizing the phenomena arising in your body and mind right now.

All actions that empty you of thoughts and emotions and calm your mind, everything that brings your wandering mind back to the here and now, can be considered a form of meditation. You can do meditation while sitting down or while walking, and you can do it while drinking a cup of tea. While you're doing it, the various thoughts and emotions that wander around your head calm down, letting you see more clearly the situation you are facing or the tasks you need to accomplish. Wisdom and insight to help you make the right choices and take the right actions well up from within a calm, clear mind. Although there are many ways to meditate, the one I use most often is breathing meditation. It is simple and easy, and its effects are powerful.

During the 60 years that constitute the first half of life, people may not have enough time to feel and watch themselves, and they have a hard time focusing on the here and now because they are dealing with the problem of making a living and because of the different forms of emotional exhaustion that come from personal relationships. But time is no longer an obstacle for elderly people, who may be bored because they don't know what they should do with all that time on their hands. For most seniors, saying "I don't have enough time to meditate" is nothing more than an excuse.

There is a lot to be gained from meditation. First of all, you can cleanse your information and control your mind through meditation. Living amid the conflicts of personal relationships and the trials of life, everyone is bound to experience a troubled heart sometimes, no matter what great, bright awakening of consciousness they have experienced. It's only natural. Meditation is an excellent way to calm agitation and to smooth out emotional ups and downs.

Think about what your breathing has been like when you've been angry, for example. Your respiration was probably short, shallow, and rough. When that happens, try sitting quietly and just controlling your breathing, without doing anything else. Simply breathe in slowly and exhale long, slow breaths. Control your breathing that way for a while and you'll find that, amazingly, the energy of anger subsides and your mind calms down. Your emotions fall away and your reason returns. You made this change just by breathing, without doing anything else at all, but surprisingly, it controls your mind. As more oxygen is supplied to your body and brain through your calm breathing, different physiological phenomena take place. Your heartbeat and brainwaves recover stability, mood-stabilizing hormones are secreted, and the muscles of your body relax. You've done breathing meditation without even realizing it.

Many studies have shown that meditation reduces stress, stabilizes the mind, and creates positive emotions. Some studies also indicate that when we meditate, physical changes occur in parts of the brain that control feelings of compassion and happiness. A research team led by Dr. Sarah Lazar, a psychologist at Harvard University Medical School, found that even ordinary people—not just meditation experts like Tibetan monks—experience a thickening of specific brain parts when they meditate. The researchers had working professionals meditate for 40 minutes a day for as little as two months or as long as a year. They discovered that the areas of the brain handling feelings of compassion and happiness grew 0.1 to 0.2 mm thicker in these people. In short, meditation helps our brains better express our spiritual potential.

Meditation also allows you to feel your soul. To live a spiritual life and to develop the energy of your soul, you must not miss the feeling of your soul. You have to know whether you are living the spiritual life that you ought to be living and whether your work, actions, and behavior have a negative or positive effect on the growth of your soul. The only standard you have to check this against is the standard of your soul. An accurate assessment is possible only if you let go of all your thoughts and feelings and go back to a state of nothingness, to zero, the original state of your soul. Meditation is the way to let go of your thoughts, emotions, and attachments so that you can once again feel your soul.

People commonly think that meditation is difficult and can only be learned with guidance from an expert. Of course, the instruction of an expert may be needed, depending on your purpose for meditating. However, I don't think meditation is difficult to practice or is separate from daily life. Just as exercise should be incorporated into your lifestyle, so too should meditation be a part of your daily life. In that sense, sleeping is the simplest and easiest form of meditation. You can get up feeling refreshed in the morning if, before going to sleep, you breathe deeply and slowly, meditating on filling your body with life energy. What's more, you can do breathing meditation even while you walk by counting your footsteps, inhaling every fourth step, and then exhaling after four more steps. You can adjust the number of your steps according to the length of your breaths. Soon you will have the amazing experience of natural life energy, along with oxygen, filling your whole body.

Breathing Meditation for Encountering the Soul

For those who are familiar with meditation, it probably won't be uncomfortable to sit in a half-lotus posture or in a chair with your back straight, but for beginners, such postures can cause tension. If that is the case, adopt a posture in which you can relax your body as much as possible, sitting with your back against a sofa or reclining with your back against a cushion. Close your eyes and slowly inhale and exhale. Now focus your mind on your chest and heart. Imagine breathing life energy into the soul in your heart.

Feel your breath gradually deepening as your body and mind relax. Forget special breathing methods and just breathe however your soul wants. You'll find a rhythm for your breathing after a while. As you inhale, imagine the life energy of the cosmos entering your body, awakening the energy of your soul in your chest. You'll feel your heart gradually filling with warmth and peace—the pure energy in your heart, the feeling of your soul. Feeling the soul is never difficult. Just let yourself be breath itself.

Breathing is a time for fully feeling your life, a time for being one with pure energy. Whenever you feel that you're mired in thought and emotion, when you feel that your life has somehow lost its center and direction, balance yourself through breathing. The goal of a spiritual life is to remain centered in your soul and to develop the strength of your soul.

Yet another advantage that can be obtained through meditation is being able to experience oneness with the life energy of the cosmos. Specifically, it's experiencing the shin, the divine energy in your brain, growing brighter. This is called a Shinmyung state.

During meditation, you can feel and see in your mind's eye the bright light of the energy of the cosmos pouring down into you and strengthening the divine energy in your brain. You'll have a feeling of integration, of being completely one with the life energy of the cosmos. You'll experience a crisp, clear insight into the principles of life or be filled with gladness, trembling, and gratitude as you receive incredible love and blessings coming from the Creator or the Source of life.

It's not easy to experience this Shinmyung state by doing breathwork just once, however. A great deal of time and effort must be committed to the practice. And for this, a little deeper, more specialized approach to breathing meditation is required. Different meditation methods are available, depending on your circumstances, and you may need the guidance of an expert for specific practices. I'll explain one briefly here.

Deeply relax by stretching your neck, shoulders, upper back, lower back, and hip joints so that your body is not tense. Sit on the floor in a half-lotus posture or in a chair. Straighten your spine and smile gently. Only then will your brain not be under pressure. Breath will enter your body comfortably only if your brain is in its most comfortable state, with your body well balanced and your spine straight.

Focus your mind in your lower abdomen, in your lower dahnjon, allowing your breath to sink deep into your belly. Your lower abdomen expands naturally when you inhale and contracts when you exhale. It helps to imagine your lower abdomen as a balloon that expands when you blow air into it and contracts when the air escapes. This is called Dahnjon Breathing.

Breathe as naturally as possible, without holding your breath, in a way that's comfortable for you. This will prevent your brain and body from tensing up. And don't lose the steady thread of your breath going in and out of your body. If you hold your breath, pull it in too hard, or let it go too quickly, that thread will break. Don't let yourself be too rushed, but don't be too slow about it, either. Concentrate only on breathing in and out, without interruption. If that thread of breath is broken, it means that distracting thoughts have entered your mind. Return your mind's eye to your body, and feel and focus on your breathing again.

Dahnjon Breathing is like lighting a fire in the energy center of the lower abdomen. Think of your dahnjon as a furnace that should always have a fire burning brightly. When the furnace heats up, the energy of your dahnjon naturally gets boiling hot. If you continue to stoke the fire by concentrating on your breathing, at some point your dahnjon will blaze red hot. Then, Water Up, Fire Down circulation arises as the water energy of the kidneys rises along the spine to cool and refresh the head. You'll develop a clear state of consciousness, free from thoughts or emotions like desire, fear, anxiety, and loneliness.

After you have breathed for a while, you may also experience different energy phenomena, such as seeing auras before your eyes. Continue watching without concerning yourself with whether your vision is dark or bright, with whatever phenomena may occur. Breathe focusing only on your dahnjon. At some moment, brilliant light—the essence of life—will appear, like a dragon rising out of deep waters. Different people experience that light in different ways. It may be a light with a specific color or form, it may be a sense of brightness, it may be a feeling that your being is transcending space and time and expanding to infinity, or it may be a sense of deep connection with some Being that feels divine and infinite. The ecstasy you will feel on encountering that light, divinity, or wholeness is indescribable. You will tremble and be deeply moved by that great love, which completely enfolds your being; it cannot be compared with love received from anyone in the world.

In this way, through deep breathing meditation, you can illuminate the shin energy and encounter the divinity within your brain. Everyone breathes. But with a proper method and intention, breathing can be a spiritual practice for encountering your soul and being one with the divine.

Meditation is a crucial element of spiritual life in old age when we head toward completion. Through meditation, you can maintain the feeling of your soul, and you can have the intense experience of being one with the energy that comes from the Source of life. That experience enables you to be certain that later, when you meet death, you will be one with the energy of the Source that you have experienced through meditation. It's not about experiencing Chunhwa when you die but about experiencing Chunhwa while you are living. Masters of the Sundo tradition, sensitive to the fact that death was approaching, consciously controlled even their final breaths. They experienced the great cycle of life as the life energy they received from the Source now returned to that Source as they slowly breathed their last.

If you already meditate, I urge you to develop your meditation into more than a tool for relieving stress, improving stability of body and mind, and increasing focus. Take it further as a means for instilling your life with the sacred by encountering your soul and becoming one with the great life force of the cosmos. If you have never meditated, I definitely suggest that you try it, setting aside the thought "That's not for me." If sitting in quiet meditation seems difficult, first do mind-body training that involves movement, such as yoga, tai chi, and kigong, so you can feel your body and develop a sense for the life energy within you. Then do meditation.

For more detail on methods of meditation for attaining Shinmyung based on Korean Sundo, I suggest that you read my books *Healing Chakras: Awaken Your Body's Energy System for Complete Health, Happiness, and Peace* and *LifeParticle Meditation: A Practical Guide to Healing and Transformation*. You can find guided video meditations in the special online course at Live120YearsCourse.com.

Never Stop Cultivating Yourself

Self-cultivation is "making yourself." It's a process of choosing who you will be and then becoming that person. To put it another way, it's a process of discovering your life and creating your own destiny. Therefore, continuous self-development is essential in the journey of a life lived in pursuit of completion.

Everyone has a creative nature and a need to realize that

creative nature. This need doesn't decrease or disappear just because we grow older. Many people actually express their creativity more actively when they're older and give themselves to self-cultivation.

You might have pursued self-development during your period of success for the purpose of improving your resume. In many cases, it has been an activity for increasing your commercial value in your field of work. During retirement, however, you can engage in self-cultivation not simply as a means to attain success, but for the pure joy and inner satisfaction that comes from working to make yourself better, for maturity of character and completion of the soul.

As long as we live, we should realize our creative nature through unending self-cultivation. We should work to renew ourselves every day until that final moment when our hearts and brains stop working. Today needs to somehow be different from yesterday, and tomorrow needs to be better than today. Stopping self-renewal is like floating in the middle of the ocean on a boat with its engine shut off.

Creativity isn't only the ability to make something new. It is also the ability to instill newness in the work we do, even if we continue in the same role. Creativity comes from curiosity and an attitude of exploration, from a questioning attitude. Ideas that can change your life and contribute to the world develop when you take a warm interest in yourself and the world. You'll get lots of ideas if, whatever environment you're in, you spend time thinking, "What can I do in this environment?" Immediately act on those ideas, even if they are small ones. Such actions come together to create change and growth in life.

Self-cultivation doesn't mean that you have to take classes from a professional to learn something new. Continuously thinking good thoughts, acting on those thoughts, and moving your body and mind are all self-development. Speaking a previously unknown language, lifting heavier weights, and handling new devices aren't the only types of results to be gained from self-development. Being able to smile more often, overlooking the mistakes of others with a smile, telling someone more easily that you love them, and being true to yourself—these are also the results of self-development.

Self-cultivation presupposes self-exploration, for you cannot truly develop and grow unless you know yourself. And true self-cultivation never ends with yourself. When you develop yourself, you find that the benefits extend to your family and other people, to your community, to your country, and to the whole planet. Changes in you lead to changes in the entire world.

Our attitude for self-cultivation in our period of completion is like that of an artist with a spirit of craftsmanship. The craftsman does his best at every moment, without using any shortcuts or tricks, to achieve a high-quality product that gives him a sense of satisfaction.

There is a famous story about Italian Renaissance artist Michelangelo when he was painting the large ceiling fresco in the Vatican's Sistine Chapel. One day, a friend saw Michelangelo in a very uncomfortable position looking up from the top of a high platform, devotedly working on every nook and cranny of the ceiling. "Look, my friend," he said, "who will ever know you so devotedly painted even that obscure corner?" "I will," Michelangelo answered.

Developing yourself with the spirit of completion is like that. It's about examining yourself honestly through contemplation and meditation, perceiving what changes are needed, choosing to create those changes, and putting your choice into action with your will. In that process, our souls become beacons on our journey toward completion. Self-cultivation in the period of completion is not something we do to compete with other people, however. If we compete with anyone, it is with the person we were yesterday.

There are all sorts of deadlines for success, but there is only one deadline for self-cultivation directed toward completion: the final moment of life.

" Meditation is a crucial element of spiritual life in old age, when we head toward completion. Through meditation, you can maintain the feeling of your soul, and you can have the intense experience of being one with the energy that comes from the Source of life."

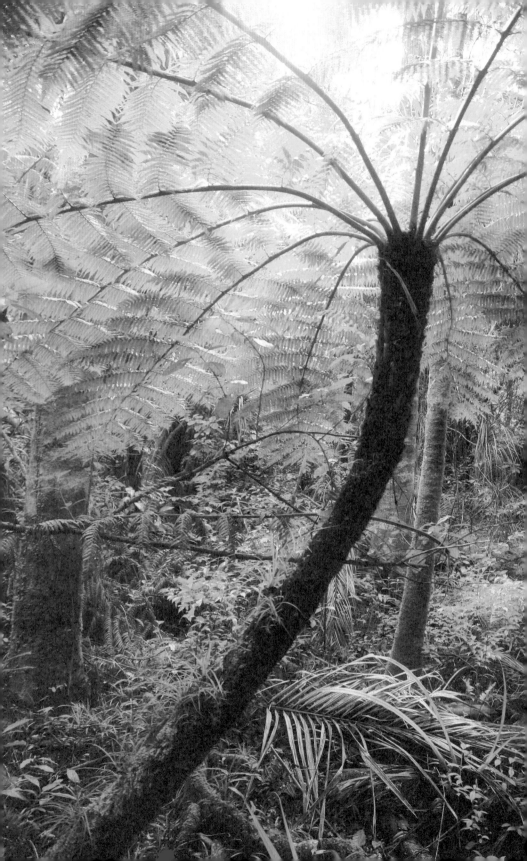

CHAPTER 11

Share and Give

The greatest regret many people have before dying, as mentioned in Chapter 2, is that they didn't have the courage to live a life true to themselves. The life you truly want, not the life others expect you to live, is a life lived true to your soul.

Did I live a life true to myself? This is the most important measure for people to use as they reflect upon their lives before death. They might be satisfied with their lives or regret their lives depending on the answer to this question. This question is like the light of wisdom guiding us in the direction we ought to travel in our old age.

People want to share the energy of the soul that they carry in their hearts. They dream of their souls becoming happier as they express and share pure love with others. Amazingly, this spring of pure love in each of our hearts never runs dry, no matter how much we use it; in fact, it grows more abundant the more we draw from it. A life lived growing our souls and helping others by sharing the energy of pure love, that is the direction of the life people who have awakened to their souls truly want.

What is the standard for living as your heart desires, without harming yourself or others? It is the standard of the growth of the soul. If you live thinking of your soul, you can never hurt yourself or others. People act rudely because they have lost their standard concerning the soul. Confucius said, "At 70, I followed my heart's desire without overstepping the boundaries of what was right." It's not easy to live a life that does no harm to others. Going a step further, though, to live helping others—not merely causing no harm—is definitely the most desirable life. That is a life of Hongik, of working for the good of all.

When you help others, the energy of your soul grows and matures. You will meet your death confidently and peacefully if your heart is contented. You cannot feel such satisfaction and peace if you have only spent your life satisfying the desires and selfishness of the ego. Many regrets will remain.

To Die without Regret

Living a life you won't regret when you die—that, I think, is the major standard we should have in our old age. That will help keep you from making choices you'll regret. We are confronted with many forks in the road and countless choices. "Should I choose this or that?" Our choices will grow easier if we ask ourselves, "When I die, will I regret the choice I'm about to make?" We can find inspiration for designing our old age by thinking, "What do I really need to do to die without regrets, with confidence that I've lived a good life?"

It is extremely important to find work that the soul in our heart truly wants us to do, not what others expect of us. We need to find the kind of work we will never regret doing but would regret never having done—that kind of work and life. Only then can we live with excitement and passion even in our later years. Passion revives when the energy of your soul fills your heart. Find the work and life that will fill your heart with passion. This is essential in order to be healthier, happier, and more peaceful.

From that perspective, I say, "For me, enlightenment is no big deal. It's just a matter of knowing what I really need." Many people who are habituated to materialism spend their time in overconsumption and waste, purchasing this and that without thinking about it much, not knowing what it is they really need. If you're someone who really knows what you need, then you will choose carefully what is essential for you. To know what you need, you have to know your true values. When you know whether you are your ego or your true self, you awaken to your true values and can make choices based on those values.

Those who realize these values put real thought into what they need to do for their growth and development, and how to live lives for their growth. The solution isn't difficult. You can design such a life if you know what you really need and know what others really need. If something is good for you and good for others, then it's ultimately good for everyone. If you help other people to become healthier, happier, and more peaceful, then you, too, will become healthier, happier, and more peaceful. The energy of joy in your heart doubles in power when you make other people smile.

Seniors who have awakened to this principle place importance on the joy and sense of reward that come through a life of service. They help the socially disadvantaged in organizations such as welfare centers for children and the elderly. They give free lectures or contribute their skills, perhaps doing someone's hair or giving music lessons. They do social work or, contributing a portion of their income, engage in charitable activities to make their communities better places to live.

Also, you'll be helping yourself as you help others. Those who do such volunteer activities, according to some studies, live much longer than those who do not. According to a study report published in the medical journal *The Lancet* in 2014, the probability of death for people with a high level of purposefulness in their lives decreased 30 percent during the eight and a half years of the study. Research into long-lived seniors around the world indicates that doing something meaningful— whether it's helping your children or volunteering in your community—has a life-extending effect of seven years.

People Who Create the Joy of Sharing

"I'm satisfied with myself right now," says Susan Gerace with a cheerful smile and shining eyes. Introduced briefly in Chapter 1, Susan didn't think that way at all five years ago when she voluntarily retired at the age of 68. She thought that she had prepared adequately for life during retirement, but upon retiring, she realized that she had been completely unprepared emotionally. She says:

> I was a nurse specializing in the newborn unit, and I had done a lot of good for patients . . . . I don't do that anymore. Who am I? Where is everyone? When I look back now, I realize that it was hard and took me a lot of time to conquer those questions and emotions. I had to find myself away from all that external stimulation and applause for the work I had been doing. To put it more precisely, I had to find a way to find myself.

The meditation Susan had been doing since before retiring and the nature retreats she regularly took part in helped her find her value inside instead of outside herself. She now does regular volunteer work at more than 10 locations, including a women's shelter, serving children from disadvantaged environments, children with special needs, and victims of domestic violence age 55 and above. She is happy and grateful whenever she sees her small acts of kindness or encouraging words having a positive effect on these people.

She maintains good relationships with her children, grandchildren, and friends of 30 years, but Susan says that she still sometimes has moments when she feels troubled and lonely. She had a crisis last year, too. For comfort, she often relied on ice cream, chocolate, an easy chair, and a TV. Thinking one day that she should change the way she was living, she gave her precious recliner to a neighbor. Surprised, the neighbor asked why—to which Susan answered, "I was sitting in it too much." She also got rid of her television, which had practically formed a set with the easy chair.

"The TV was always on. But that doesn't mean I always watched it. The TV was filling an empty house where there was no one but me." It took several weeks until she was able to get by without the television and easy chair. "I can do this," she kept telling herself. "I can do this." It really took courage.

Having activities that give meaning to life in old age will help you in many ways, Susan says. For her, those activities include helping people in difficult environments and sharing fulfilling life experiences with her family. Although getting rid of her recliner and TV provided an opportunity for change, other daily activities she had always done—like meeting with family and doing volunteer work—brought her renewed vitality and enabled her to escape from her habitual loneliness. The meditation she likes best these days is watching a beautiful sunrise or sunset over the Arizona desert. Every time she does this, she feels intense peace and a strong connection with all life.

"Aging well is accepting yourself just as you are. And I think that it includes drawing closer to and helping others as well as yourself," says Susan.

Seventy-six this year, Janet Duda retired at the age of 67 after working as a nurse for 43 years. She thought a lot about how to remain healthy and happy while caring for elderly patients who suffered from depression, anxiety disorder, and dementia. Before retiring, she and her husband set up a plan and prepared for retirement life. As soon as she retired, they toured the United States for three and a half years in a 32-foot trailer; occasionally they traveled to more distant places, such as Europe. Since settling in Las Vegas in 2010, she has been volunteering in their local community.

Janet volunteers at an animal shelter for five hours every Saturday, helping with puppy adoptions, walking and hugging the dogs, and doing laundry. She also works at a shelter for victims of domestic abuse. She uses her truck to transport donated furniture. She once delivered a bed set to a family that had been sleeping on the floor or a sofa for a month. The family was so happy that they hugged her 14 times and later sent her a message telling her it had been the best Christmas gift ever. In addition, Janet volunteers at a police station, where her job is to role-play for new recruits or students at the police academy. She has played a variety of roles, from domestic violence victim to drunk driver, and even someone in possession of a weapon. Janet has been actively volunteering at her temple, too. This is what she says:

> Fortunately, my profession, nursing, was itself a life of helping people. Possibly for that reason, I got addicted to helping other people. It makes you feel good to know that you've made a difference in someone's life. I need it like I need food and drink. If I wasn't doing this, I would be sad and lonely. I'm a firm believer that everyone needs something to get them up and excited

in the morning. In order to feel good, it's important to have something to look forward to doing, and especially to feel happy about what you're doing. I don't do things I don't like.

I know that death is coming for me, too, and that I've come more than halfway down the road to death. I think that something is waiting after this life, although I don't know what it is. And I believe that this life isn't the end. When the time comes, I feel like this has been a good life. I feel like I've made a difference in some lives, and that's good. I'm content with that.

How Should I Use My Life Energy?

What could be more satisfying than using the precious time and energy called "life" to somehow contribute to other people and the world before you die? If, instead, you let the time go by meaninglessly, wouldn't you regret it before you died? You would likely think, "I failed to make good use of the energy of love inside me."

There is a way to check how much you've grown your soul in this world before you die: by getting a sense for the feeling within your heart. The energy of your soul has grown a great deal if you feel joy and satisfaction filling your heart, and you think, "I've lived well. I'm proud of myself. Though I die now, I have no regrets in my life." But if your heart feels hollow, you haven't filled it with the energy of your soul.

You can retire from your job, but you can't retire from life—not until you die. Your life doesn't end just because you've retired from your job. Life is the precious time and the physical power, heart power, and brain power you've been given. Whether it came from the God who created this world or the Source of the great life of the cosmos, the right to use that life energy was transferred to you the moment you were born. That right was given only to you, until you die. You're the only one who can decide how to use it. Your life energy doesn't want to be wasted meaninglessly. It wants to be used for meaningful things, for making people and the world healthier, happier, and more peaceful.

While you live, you are the master of that life energy. Will you put it to good use as its true master, or will you be a spectator, standing by and watching with your arms folded? A life as master or a life as spectator—you must choose between the two. Find and design what you really want to achieve so you'll be free of regrets at the moment of death.

Ask yourself, "If I knew that today was the last day of my life, would I go ahead with what I had planned for the day?" If you think you would, then what you are doing now is clearly meaningful. But if not, find what it is that your soul really wants to do. I want to cheer you on, hoping you will be able to discover something that fills you with excitement and passion, something you won't regret though you die doing it, something you would gladly do even on the last day of your life. What you vividly dream becomes reality!

" A life lived growing our souls
and helping others by sharing
the energy of pure love, that is
the direction of the life people
who have awakened to their
souls truly want."

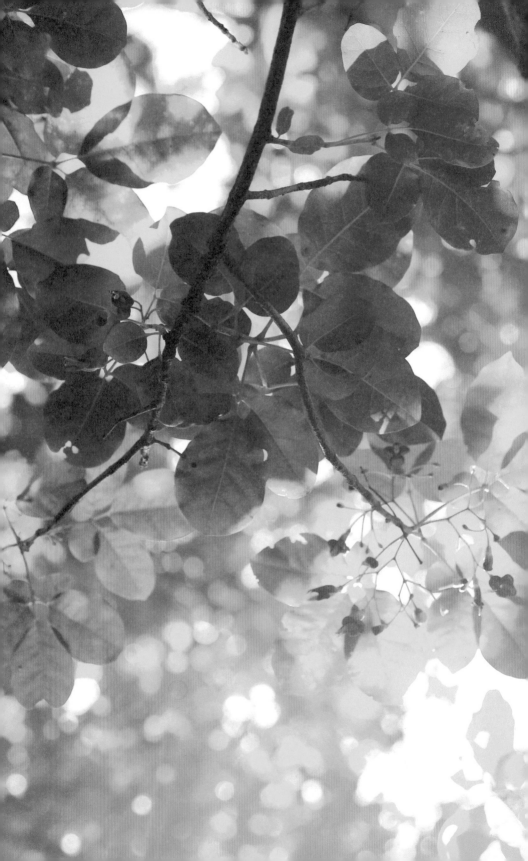

CHAPTER 12

Be Close to Nature

In old age, I think it's best to live where you can get closer to nature than you can in a busy city. If that's not possible, then visit natural places often, wherever you may be and whenever you get the chance. You don't necessarily have to go to distant mountains or the wilderness, or to the ocean. A park or trail near your home is good, too—wherever you can feel the sunshine, trees, water, and wind, wherever you can see the open sky and walk on unpaved ground.

Getting close to nature is a wonderful way to fill our lives with spirituality and a sense of completion. To understand why, you must first realize the character of the relationship between you and nature. I have experienced that process of realization, and it happened in three phases.

About 20 years ago, when I first visited Sedona, Arizona, a place surrounded by red earth and majestic rock formations and carpeted with a lush green forest of cactuses and juniper trees, I thought of nothing but enjoying the beautiful scenery. Bewitched by Sedona's intense, mysterious charm, I was continuously awestruck by the surrounding beauty. "I can't believe there is somewhere on earth so beautiful!" I repeated to myself as I made my way around Sedona.

But at some moment, I realized that before I was watching Sedona, Sedona was watching me! Yes, the red rocks, cactuses, and junipers of Sedona had existed there long before me, watching multitudes come and go. I was but one of those many people. We humans are here for a moment, I felt, and then we are gone. The true master of this land was none other than nature herself.

I had another realization in that same moment: I am a part of nature. Nature and I are one whole, not separate things. Why am I nature? I am an organism living and breathing in the massive ecosystem of the earth. The realization that I am one with nature felt powerful, like rolling thunder. That awakening shook my whole body, my very cells. It is no exaggeration to say that this is the beginning and the end of enlightenment.

The truth is simple: humans and nature are one. From a certain point of view, this is a common sense notion that even children know. The problem is that people usually know this only with their heads, as a kind of intellectual knowledge. To really understand it, we must experience it throughout all the cells in our bodies, as a feeling that is more than knowledge. When you really feel that you're one with nature, you can experience a great integration of consciousness wherein you are interconnected with everything you once perceived as separate from yourself.

If you wish to spend your old age aiming for spiritual completion, grow as close to nature as possible. This cannot be overstated.

Let Go of Your Ego

A nature-friendly life helps you let go of your ego.

If you dig deeply into the fundamental reasons people are so troubled and suffer so much, you will discover that it is because of their egos. The word ego signifies the false identity that an individual holds, the self that appears to exist separately from nature and others. From the perspective of the ego, you see yourself as an individual separate from the whole. When caught up in this sense of self, you experience the anguish and endless conflict that come from incompleteness.

Buddhists believe that people are kept from escaping the ego, a state known as nirvana, by three poisons: greed, anger, and foolishness. Greed is the desire to fill our incompleteness through material gain or something from outside; anger arises when our greed is not satisfied; and foolishness is the failure to act according to the knowledge that we are all one.

The problem is separation consciousness—the thought that you and I are separate, that nature and I are separate. This dualistic worldview, which perceives the individual ego as subject and everything else, even nature, as objects separate from self, is at the root of most problems on this planet. For people continuously educated to perceive self and others as separate and accustomed to chasing the paradigm of success— which tells us to compete, own, and control as much as possible in a materialistic society—the desires of the ego have an increasingly powerful effect as time goes on. And the more that happens, the more people become mired in pain. People have even made the earth and sky sick by perceiving humanity as something separate from nature, viewing it merely as a resource to be exploited and developed. Our pollution of the sky and ground is finally coming back to haunt us, and it's making people sick. How can we fix this?

The solution, once you understand it, is clear. The problem has been the worldview that sees everything as separate, so what we have to do is switch to a holistic worldview that sees everything as one. Changing the entire social system—things like education, politics, economics, and culture—will take a great deal of time and effort. Our consciousness as individuals, though, can change right now.

There is an easy way to let go of the ego and have a holistic perspective: feel that you are one with nature. The ego is really tough and tenacious. It's useless to try to rip out your ego forcibly; turn around, and you'll find it right back where it was. Though you resolve every day to set aside your ego, before you know it, the ego will revive as you are harassed by trouble with work and relationships in your daily life. However, the ego usually falls away in the instant you feel oneness with nature. That becomes possible when you feel nature with every cell in your body, not just understand her as a bit of knowledge.

Open your body and mind while surrounded by the energies of Heaven and earth. Feel the breath of nature, and experience interconnection with the energy of nature. When you feel that you are a part of nature—a part of the life energy field of the whole—the separation consciousness of the ego vanishes on its own, and great awakening comes. You will be able to say with sincerity, "I am one with nature." But saying this while you still cling to your ego is incomplete. The realization has to go deeper, through feeling rather than thought. That's why you need to meditate in nature.

You've probably already experienced that you can escape from your ego quickly when you get close to nature. Have you ever laced up your sneakers to go for a walk when your mind was a tangle of thoughts and emotions, then breathed out the frustration in your heart as you enjoyed a pleasant breeze beneath a brightly shining sun? If you walk a few dozen minutes like that, your roiling thoughts and emotions soon quiet down, and your mind grows brighter and lighter. Reality hasn't changed at all, but the world looks different because your mind and your energy have changed. Nature has an amazing power to purify the energy of our thoughts and emotions, returning us to our original, natural state.

Befriend Nature

A nature-friendly life allows us to befriend nature.

We grow close to as well as distant from many friends as we live our lives. How many of the people with whom we promised undying friendship during our school years do we find around us in our old age? Approaching death, many people count their failure to stay in touch with friends as one of their principal regrets. Close friends in youth unintentionally lose contact as they become immersed in their separate lives. If you have even one true friend you can share your heart with, rely on, and get help from when things are hard, then you can say that you have lived a good life. Life situations, environments, thoughts, and emotions can make relationships difficult to maintain. Wouldn't it be great if you had a friend who fully knew your heart, with whom you could communicate on a heart-to-heart level? The loneliness of old age, when we are left alone after our friends and loved ones have left the world one by one, is difficult to endure.

Let's not just lament that we're alone and lonely in our old age. We simply have to make new friends. The depth and affection we experience may be less than with old companions, but we can still meet and share our hearts with new friends as we grow old together. And remember, we have one lifelong friend who can be with us to the very end: nature.

From a certain perspective, nature may feel far more comfortable as a friend than another person does. Each of us has a framework of experiences, personality traits, and ideas that form as we live our lives. Personal relationships are a process of learning a harmony that embraces even the differences between people. But it can be uncomfortable when such differences put us in conflict, so we end up avoiding spending time with people. With nature, though, we don't need to worry about those clashes. Why? Because nature doesn't judge us. She accepts and embraces us just as we are. She's a warm refuge we can rely on for rest when things get tough, an affectionate friend who encourages us and tells us to have hope and courage.

Everyone has probably had the experience of being loved

and comforted by nature. When we sit in warm sunshine on a bright spring day or lie on the grass looking up at the sky, when we walk a woodland trail listening to bird songs, when we look out over the open sea and feel refreshed, when we gaze up at the stars twinkling in the inky darkness—in these moments we smile and say to nature, "Wow . . . that's beautiful." Our hearts open up as if we've just met an old friend. When we open our hearts, we can hear what nature is saying to us. "Have courage! It's all right. You can do it! I love you." Those messages are actually voices echoing within us; the nature inside us has revived. When the nature within and the nature without are connected as one, we can hear its messages. Then we become the true friends of nature.

Friendship is not unilateral, but a mutual exchange. To be a friend of nature, you must be able to sympathize with it, not just enjoy its beauty. You have to open your heart to nature, just as you open your heart to befriend another human being. When we open up, nature comes into our hearts, and the naturalness within us revives because of nature's energy of pure love. Then we say, "I am nature" and "I am one with nature."

Where could we find another friend like nature with whom we can be completely open? Nature is there beside you, the greatest and most intimate of friends. Nature watches without emotion or judgment and accepts you fully. She is someone with whom you can have wholehearted communion. Oh, you seniors who have endured difficult lives, find comfort in nature. It will heal the wounds you've suffered and open your closed heart.

In Korea long ago, learned men would retire from the world to live simple, contented lives in nature, and they would sing songs like this:

The verdant mountains are my friends,
    as are the green trees.
The wind and moon between the verdant mountains
    and green trees are also my friends.
I will grow old with these four beauties
    for the rest of my life.
    —Author unknown

You ask how many friends I have?
Water and rock, pine and bamboo.
I'm even gladder to see the moon rising
    above the eastern hill.
Let me be. What would I do with more friends
    than these five?
    —From "Song of Five Friends" by Seondo Yun

Be Charged with Complete Energy

Yet another advantage of a nature-friendly life is that it allows us to be completely charged with energy from nature.

We can live only if we receive energy, because we are organisms made up of energy. The food we eat is an energy source used to maintain the life energy of our bodies. But we need energy for our souls as well as energy for our bodies. People thirst for energy that can enrich their souls and give them new inspiration. To receive such energy, they pursue personal relationships, feel a sense of achievement through work, have hobbies, or engage in spiritual or religious life. Although such activities comfort their hearts to some degree, there are many times when they don't feel fully satisfied.

We pursue completeness or wholeness. Our lives are spent wandering in search of wholeness, of something that can satisfy us completely. But wholeness is not found in the artificial. Wholeness exists only in nature. Nature itself is wholeness. Of course, we can be made whole, too, because we are nature—that is, if we contain the fullness of nature within us.

Try setting everything aside and lying down for a moment in the bosom of nature. Your body and soul will be filled by the warm sunshine, fresh air, crisp sound of running water, and refreshing smell of grass and soil. Nature always sends us the energy of infinite love and blessings, a complete energy that humans cannot fabricate. If you want to obtain perfect energy, let yourself be charged with the infinite energy of nature. The wholeness that has always been within you will revive in that instant.

We have physical parents who gave birth to us and raised us, but we also have greater parents who supported our lives through the whole process of being conceived, being born, and growing up. These are our cosmic parents. The food and water that enter our bodies through our mouths are the energy we get from the earth; air and sunshine are energy we get from the heavens. The human organism could not survive for even 10 minutes without the energy of the heavens and the earth. We can live right now, breathing and active, because we have nature, our cosmic parents. Just as physical parents give their sacrificial love to their children, our cosmic parents give humanity their unconditional love—and they demand nothing in exchange for that love. If there is one thing that our cosmic parents want from us, it is that we live in harmony with all creatures on the planet, just as physical parents want their children to get along well with one another.

Do you need energy? Don't just seek it from other people; be filled with the life energy of nature, our cosmic parents. Nature fills your body with a life energy that instills vitality in your soul so that your heart pulses with joy. That is a complete, perfect energy of peace you cannot get from anyone else.

Fill yourself with nature, and don't forget to share with those around you the energy you have received from nature. Getting love from nature and sharing it with others, sharing unconditional love just as nature does, that is the life of a natural person.

Prepare to Return to Nature

A nature-friendly life prepares us to return to the bosom of nature after death.

Nature doesn't speak; it merely shows us things as they are. The way for us to become one with nature is to feel nature as it is. We can commune with nature through the meditation of silence. Nature contains truths inexpressible in speech or writing, and we are deeply moved when we feel that. The same is true with humans; we are moved more by someone's character and integrity than by his or her words. It is a tremendous blessing that humans have a sense for detecting truth beyond the spoken and written word. The life of a natural person is about keeping that sense alive.

Nature is our teacher. She is the common teacher of all humankind, a teacher who is always close by, one we can meet anytime and anywhere, and who holds immutable truths. We learn wisdom and life principles through nature. We awaken to the principles of nature in the cycles of spring, summer, fall, and winter. We discover in the brilliant sun great love shining equally on everyone, and we feel the wonder of life in new shoots and flowering petals.

Students tend to resemble their teachers, so the closer to nature humans become, the more their character resembles nature. More and more, they resemble the virtue of the immense expanses of the earth, which embraces and nurtures all life, and the wisdom of the boundless heavens, which provide light, freedom, and peace. If, as you grow older, your character becomes more like that of nature, you will experience oneness with nature with your whole body. Humans, it is said, came from nature and return to nature. We prepare to return to the bosom of nature, prepare to experience Chunhwa, becoming one with Heaven.

The amazing wisdom and principles of nature are contained in the 81 characters of the Chun Bu Kyung, Korea's oldest scripture.

Il Shi Mu Shi Il (一始無始一)
Bon Shim Bon Tae Yang Ang Myung (本心本太陽昂明)
In Joong Chun Ji Il (人中天地一)
Il Jong Mu Jong Il (一終無終一)

Everything begins in One,
but that One is without beginning.
The original mind, bright like the sun, pursues brightness.
Heaven and earth are one in humanity.
Everything ends in One, but that One is without end.

This is the key passage from the Chun Bu Kyung. It means that the eternity of the cosmos and nature is One without beginning and without end. We should pursue the original mind, which is bright like the sun, and awaken to the oneness of nature (the heavens and the earth) within us. Awakening to this principle and pursuing a life based on it is a life of preparing for completion of the soul, for Chunhwa.

Growing to resemble nature and being one with nature is an ideal that anyone would dream of for their old age. Whether we are born in a rich home or a poor one, we are all similar when we get old and face death, even if we once had amazing wealth, power, or intellect. All are equal before nature. So setting aside the burden of our power, prestige, greed, and attachments to become people of nature is the right attitude to have when preparing for death. It's all about fine-tuning your energy—making it brighter, freer, and more peaceful—as you prepare to return to the fundamental life energy of the cosmos.

As long as your life energy remains, you can lovingly embrace all people and all life with an open heart. Sharing our time on planet Earth is the path of the enlightened elder, the path of Chunhwa. Let us each hope that on our final day in this world, we can close our eyes in peace and contentment, and say, as this poem does, "I lived a great life."

> *Today is a very good day to die.*
> *Every living thing is in harmony with me.*
> *Every voice sings a chorus within me.*
> *All beauty has come to rest in my eyes.*
> *All bad thoughts have departed from me.*
> *Today is a very good day to die.*
> *My land is peaceful around me.*
> *My fields have been turned for the last time.*
> *My house is filled with laughter.*
> *My children have come home.*
> *Yes, today is a very good day to die.*
> —From *Many Winters* by Nancy Wood, 1974

“ Getting close to nature is a wonderful way to fill our lives with spirituality and a sense of completion. Nature has an amazing power to purify the energy of our thoughts and emotions, returning us to our original, natural state."

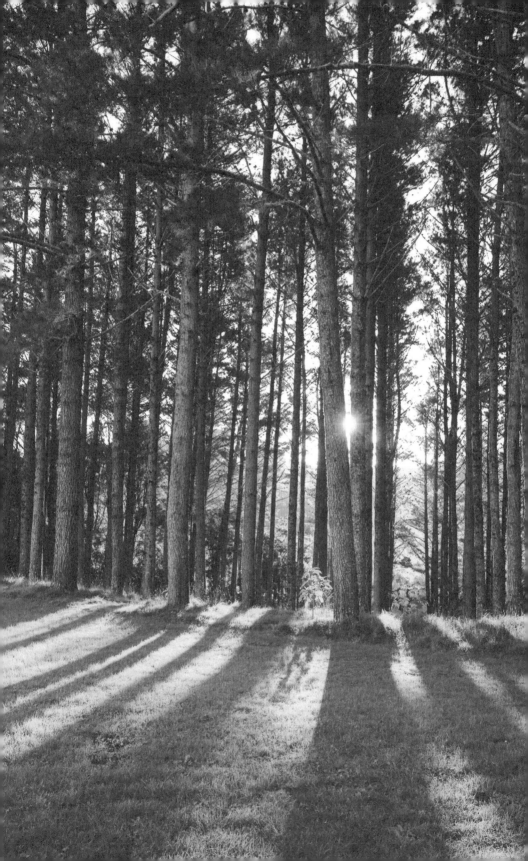

CHAPTER 13

What We Leave
Behind

I believe that the world can change for the better if we live the second half of our lives well. Life in old age holds an important key for solving many problems in our society and for ushering in a new age. We can find this possibility in the rapid growth of the older population, which is increasing the importance of senior culture and lifestyles throughout society. To put it another way, the elderly are becoming the center of society. As their share of the population grows, seniors will not only become targets for various consumer and cultural industries, but their voices will receive more attention politically and socially.

The social impact of the older generation will inevitably grow with time, so the direction in which that influence is applied is important. Will it upgrade or downgrade society? One thing will determine the answer to this question: the consciousness of elderly people. Seniors can help develop our society in innovative ways, or they can simply increase the burden on the generations supporting them. That's why I believe that a revolution in the consciousness of seniors and the emergence of enlightened elders are absolutely essential.

I am convinced that a revolution in consciousness centered on the elderly is possible. A new culture of aging could be the solution for overcoming many problems of modern society. This culture would be one in which seniors awaken to realize that their substance is life energy and that self and other, people and nature—all of us—are interconnected as one. They would make completion the goal of their lives and have lifestyles directed to that end. As the number of enlightened elders grows, the more human consciousness will develop synergy and the more likely it will be that we can change direction toward a spiritual civilization centered on completion.

Mentors for the Next Generation

In traditional societies, enlightened elders were repositories of knowledge—like an encyclopedia or a library. The wisdom and experience that older people accumulated throughout their lives was considered precious back when the pace of social change was slower than in modern societies. The elderly were respected as leaders in their villages. Elders were asked about many things: when it's best to sow seed, for example; how to teach a willful son; what to give a mother suffering from a stomach ailment; how conflicts with neighboring villages could be resolved. They were educators and healers, arbitrators and communicators, transmitting culture and wisdom from one generation to the next. Such roles maintained the values of their communities, granted stability, and brought balance.

It is no exaggeration to say that ancient thought was formed by the wisdom of the elders. The name of Laotzu, author of *Tao Te Ching*, said to have been translated into more languages than any book except the Bible, literally means Old Master. The Buddha lived to be 80 and Confucius to be 73, teaching students and sharing their wisdom with the world. Plato continued to write until he passed away at the age of 81.

Unfortunately, we find few traces today of elders sharing their wisdom as honored mentors. Young people no longer ask questions of the elderly; they ask the Internet. Older people have to learn from young people how to use smartphones and operate new devices. Younger generations often think of seniors as stubborn people who have fallen behind the times and with whom communication is difficult. Seniors who have life experiences and wisdom to share have a hard time communicating with younger generations, who instead chase after speed and sensual stimulation.

The elders of old who acted as mentors to young people should be emulated once again. But first, the consciousness of seniors must awaken. Older people can act as mentors because they have something more than informational knowledge to share. Young people have easy access to facts; they want to hear deep wisdom from those who have lived before them. They need heartwarming and refreshing words that help them see the problems they have been anguishing over from a different perspective. Younger generations need tolerant, benevolent love that can warm their increasingly cold hearts.

Such changes must happen, first and foremost, in each of

our families. We must develop a worthy family culture, one in which grandmothers and grandfathers embrace their children and grandchildren with love and lead them with wisdom. The character of children who have grown up seeing their parents respect their grandparents, who have grown up in the loving arms of their grandparents, can never be corrupted. Such children don't need to go to some private institute or organization to receive character education. Family members need to be the people who provide it.

However, the wisdom of the elderly must not remain only within the family. It should spread to the community, too. The wisdom of our seniors will never become a driving force for change if it is only used privately. It must also be used as a social resource for the larger good. For that to happen, individual seniors and society at large must work together.

Individually, seniors must have compassion and take an active interest in the affairs of the world instead of turning their backs, considering themselves old fogies who are out of sight and out of mind. They need to accept old age as an opportunity for maturity and for the completion of life. They should pursue the joy and passion that comes from helping people around them and their communities. This kind of life promotes the completion of the whole, not just the individual, and we need more people who feel that such a life is what their souls enjoy most. A society with many older people who sincerely care for their communities and who work to make the world a better place is a blessed society. If seniors gather the wisdom and experience they have built up over their lives and work for the common good, it will have a positive effect on all areas of society, including politics, economics, culture, and education.

Socially, seniors ought to be provided with abundant opportunities to share their wisdom and skills while being respected as precious members of their communities. When it comes to senior citizens' welfare, there are varying opinions. What is certain, though, is that people who are always stressed and worried about where they will get their next meal have a hard time pursuing spiritual maturity or living lives devoted to serving others.

As a society, we should look after and protect our elderly, ensuring that their basic needs are met. Caring for the elderly, however, is about more than providing meals, building senior centers, or sending social workers. Society must provide work that allows seniors to contribute to the community while feeling joy and a sense of reward. Money-making careers may end at retirement, but there are many jobs that seniors can do better than younger people.

Let's Leave Behind a Better Environment

Living life for the value of completion, not just for the value of success, is urgently needed for the protection of the global environment.

When you look at weather forecasts in Korea, you find something unique, different from what you see in the United States and other countries. The forecaster predicts the day's weather by saying that the concentration of fine dust in the air will be good, average, bad, or very bad, along with cloudy or clear. On days when fine dust is very bad, you should refrain from going out, if possible, or you should wear a special fine-dust mask. When you go out on those days, your eyes hurt, and your throat becomes sore in no time.

According to a joint 10-year study by environmental research institutes in South Korea, China, and Japan, since 2000, some 30 to 50 percent of the fine dust in Korea has blown over from China, and since 2013, this pollution has gotten worse. Fine dust caused by the accelerating industrialization of China, which depends on coal for about 70 percent of its energy, is crossing borders and polluting the atmosphere of surrounding nations.

In June 2017, citing a report by a research team at Plymouth University in the United Kingdom, the British daily *The Guardian* reported that plastic fragments had been detected in a third of the seafood caught in UK waters. Scientists at Ghent University in Belgium recently calculated that people who regularly eat seafood ingest up to 11,000 tiny pieces of plastic every year.

Those fragments come from bottles made with polyethylene (PET). When fish eat PET bottles discarded in the ocean and we eat those fish, it's as if we are eating the bottles. Even now, 1.2 million PET bottles are being sold every minute. More than 480 billion plastic drinking bottles were sold in 2016 around the world, and by 2021, this will jump another 20 percent to 583.3 billion. If the bottles that have been sold until now were placed end-to-end, they would extend more than halfway to the sun. Moreover, by 2050, the ocean will contain more plastic by weight than fish, according to research by the Ellen MacArthur Foundation. The plastic bottles that we use and discard with no thought other than convenience are threatening our dinner tables. Furthermore, rarely can we eat any agricultural or livestock products today without danger from environmental pollution, indiscriminate use of chemical products, and genetic manipulation.

The source of human life is nature. When nature gets sick, humans cannot avoid getting sick, too. Human diseases caused by environmental pollution are increasing at a rapid pace worldwide. David Pimentel, professor emeritus in the Department of Ecology and Evolutionary Biology at Cornell University, and a team of researchers from the university's graduate school announced that 40 percent of deaths around the globe are the result of polluted water, air, and soil. These findings were based on a study of more than 120 published papers on the effects of population growth, malnutrition, and environmental pollution on human disease.

The idea of humans enjoying a 120-year lifespan is nothing but fantasy unless the earth's environment becomes healthier. In the country of Chad in Africa, life expectancy is no more than 49 years because of disease, malnutrition, and a shortage of clean water. We must work simultaneously to take care of our communities and to take care of ourselves and our families. And we must care for the ecosystem of the earth itself, or the environment will reach a state from which it cannot recover. If that happens, even human survival will be difficult.

Three years ago, I shared a long conversation with Dr. Emanuel Pastreich, a scholar of East Asian studies, about what we can do to live more mindful, sustainable lives. He introduced me to the words of American environmental activist Gus Speth:

> I used to think that top environmental problems were biodiversity loss, ecosystem collapse, and climate change. I thought that 30 years of good science could address these problems. I was wrong. The top environmental problems are selfishness, greed, and apathy, and to deal with these we need a cultural and spiritual transformation. And we scientists don't know how to do that.

I fully agree that human selfishness, greed, and apathy are at the heart of our environmental problems. We must now transcend the value of success and head toward the value of completion. People who have separation consciousness based on materialism view nature as nothing more than an object to be developed and exploited for success. This is at the root of what is damaging the environment, and it makes us apathetic about that damage. Our only hope is to transcend our separation consciousness, realize that we are all one with nature, and understand fully that nature is the source of every one of our lives. When people realize these things, change will begin.

A narrow-minded perspective that thinks of only me, my

family, and my country cannot resolve the problems we are experiencing. We have to start thinking of everything as one; separation is no longer feasible. The world is not a collection of separate things; everything is interconnected by energy. We are connected by air, water, wind, and sunlight. We share everything in the global environment. No nation can stop the flow of energy by building high walls on its borders. A nation's efforts to be strong by building high walls and making regulations will backfire if its neighbors are poor and unhappy. Powerful police and piles of money cannot stop viruses or pollution from being carried in on water and wind.

If we see things from a different perspective beyond separation and our own immediate convenience and profit, we find wisdom that can solve many pressing issues of today. For example, when we stop food waste, we take a big step toward ending hunger. By some estimates, nearly half of the food grown, processed, and transported in the United States goes to waste. Every year, we spend about $1.7 trillion globally on armies, equivalent to about $247 for each of the 7 billion people in the world. If we can reduce the tremendous resources spent on armed forces and use them instead to protect the natural environment and recover the damage we have caused to nature, we can leave clearer skies and cleaner waters to the coming generations and other life forms on our planet.

If humans go on living as they are, causing massive harm to fellow humans and other organisms while thinking only of external expansion, increased human lifespan will not necessarily be a blessing for the planet. The older generation, as the enlightened elders of our time, has a responsibility to work to ensure that the way they live in their old age will improve life on the planet. Otherwise, we are just increasing the amount we take from the earth without giving anything in return.

Let's Live as Earth Citizens

I have long taught people about the Earth Citizen Spirit. The heart of that spirit is simple. It's the notion that we should live with consideration for our planet because, before we are members of any specific country, race, or religion, we are citizens of the earth. Although we have different skin colors and use different languages, there is a common denominator linking us all—we are part of a single human species living on the planet called Earth.

Not long ago, I was incredibly glad to hear Facebook founder and CEO Mark Zuckerberg, in a Harvard commencement speech, talking about the concept of being citizens of the world. If leaders like Zuckerberg who have significant social influence talk widely about the spirit of earth citizenship and continue to create global solidarity, we will be able to create positive, meaningful change.

Everyone on the planet should live with an awareness of earth citizenship. Brave environmental activists who demonstrate and take risks to stop oil spills or nuclear testing are not the only ones living as Earth Citizens. Mothers and fathers who cook and clean their homes for their families, professionals who work hard at their companies, grandmothers and grandfathers who cultivate vegetable gardens and raise chickens in the country—all of them can be Earth Citizens.

We must gain the understanding that the earth is our home, that it is ours. Let's say that you bought a car you'd been looking at for a long time, and somebody made a long scratch on it with a nail. Naturally you would be angry, disgusted, and disappointed. If someone were to try to hurt your child, you'd become braver and more powerful than the protagonist of a superhero movie. You probably wouldn't react that way if that car or child had nothing to do with you, but since it's your car and your child, you want to protect them, no matter what. We need to have that same attitude about the earth. The planet is your home. And other humans, animals, and plants are your family, beings who share the same home, this earth.

The first step for a good Earth Citizen's life is to have hope and ownership of your life. Those who have no sense of ownership or who have lost hope for their own lives will have the same kind of thinking about the planet. "Somebody else will solve the planet's problems; our leaders or experts will do the right thing," they may passively think. Or they may pessimistically think, "Nothing about the world will change no matter what anyone does." People who lack faith in themselves naturally find it difficult to have faith and hope in others and in the world.

If you feel that you are one with nature and become the true master of your life, you cannot help but develop a sense of urgency, knowing that the problems of the earth and the human species are your own. If you have a desire to help the planet and its inhabitants, even in little ways, you can make a difference. You can use your knowledge, money, power, talent, and time to benefit other people and your community. If we each give ourselves hope, we can become the hope of the earth. A new path will open up for the earth and the human race when a new path opens up in each of our lives.

Each of us has the heart of an Earth Citizen. Everyone is born with a desire for the health and happiness of other people and other life forms. We have a natural desire to contribute, even if only a little, to making a better world. Acting on that desire in our daily lives is the lifestyle of an Earth Citizen. It's the desire to pick up trash that has fallen on the street because it's the same as my own house being messy. Earth Citizens do more than just clean up their own front yards.

Your Earth Citizen mindset and your ability to act will become more powerful when they result from spontaneous realization arising within you rather than persuasive arguments made by someone else. Earth Citizens tell themselves, "The source of my life is nature. The place I've come from and the place I will return to is nature." Earth citizenship is the awareness that we should actively preserve nature and leave it to our descendants in good shape. Acting on that awareness is the responsibility of enlightened elders seeking to leave a valuable gift for the next generation.

We have come to this earth, and we need to raise and care for more than our immediate biological families. We must also care for our communities, our planet, and nature. As seniors, let us awaken and act to ensure that our earth home is safer, and let's enable our families here to be happier, too. If our descendants also wake up and follow our example, that will be even better.

Earth Citizen Hanabuchi Keiko

Hanabuchi Keiko, now 84 years old, showed me what it is to be a beautiful Earth Citizen. Until the age of 60, she worked as an instructor of English at the Japanese high school she once attended. After retiring, she took care of her mother, who had dementia; her husband, who suffered from lung cancer; and her son, who had suffered a stroke.

The year she turned 73, she occasionally took a yoga class because it was frustrating to stay all day in the hospital where her son had been admitted. One day, she learned of a Body & Brain Yoga Center that taught the mind-body training methods I had developed. Hanabuchi came to love Body & Brain Yoga training. It was a joy to get up every morning, she said, and it felt like she was living life again.

Eventually, she wanted to share her joy with others, so she opened a Body & Brain Yoga Center when she was in her mid-70s. It took her an hour and 20 minutes to get to the center from her home, but she couldn't wait to rise each morning. She cleaned the road and steps in front of the center with her own hands every morning, thinking about the people she would teach that day. Her center was very successful, thanks to her devotion and passion.

Now, a decade later, Hanabuchi has entrusted the operation of the center to someone else and is running a Happy Brain Club, a gathering for mind-body exercises that meets regularly at various places. At one time, she ran 13 such clubs. She now teaches classes at six locations.

Whatever happens, she doesn't rest from this work. If her personal situation keeps her from making a class, she always reschedules it. As few as five to as many as 15 people from their 50s to their 70s come to Hanabuchi's classes. Occasionally, she teaches at a child welfare center as well. Sometimes, young mothers bring along their children, three or four years old. She says it's a great joy to watch the kids—who call her Hanabuchi Sensei—as they do the movements she's teaching their mothers. Hanabuchi said:

Sometimes, after we're done with the training, I'll talk about the things I've learned in my life so far. It's nothing special. I teach that we need to consider the time and life we've been given as precious, and we should live doing our best, being grateful for every moment. We must develop our talents and wisdom as much as we can and use them in a way that helps others and society, as well as ourselves. People old and young think carefully about my words, sometimes even taking down notes. That's when I feel a sense of reward, thinking, "Ah, that person gets it!"

I asked Hanabuchi what she thought happy old age looked like, and this was her answer:

There is a TV drama that depicted the life of a Japanese samurai. The mother of the drama's protagonist talks about the spirit of the samurai to her son as she looks at the red autumn leaves in a field. "Do you know why autumn leaves are so beautiful? The trees are storing up energy to make it through the harsh winter. The autumn leaves are dying instead of the tree. They say that those blazing colors are the colors of resolution to defend what is more precious than one's own life."

As I watched that scene, I, too, thought that I should spend the rest of my life burning my energy up like those leaves, living for values I think are precious. Now that I'm older, everyone who passes me on the street seems like my child. When I see young children, they all seem so cute and precious, whether I know them or not. I came to the earth first and have lived longer than them, so I want to work to the very last to live a life that will allow me to say, "This is the pride and dignity of living as a human being."

Hanabuchi feels that all the people she passes on the street are her children. Having come to the earth first and having lived longer, she wants to burn with passion to the very end to protect what is precious for the community of earth. Her story inspires us to age happily and beautifully and to live as an Earth Citizen should. It's a beautiful testimony that brings a smile to my face when I hear it.

A Culture of Tolerance and Sharing

Through the first half of our individual lives, we experience how destructive it can be to pursue only possessions, control, and conquest. It is the responsibility of the senior generation to share that wisdom so it can become the guiding wisdom of all society. By teaching the values of completion to young people still in their period of success, we can prevent human life and nature from being spiritually impoverished.

Seniors can help restore balance by instilling values of sharing and giving in a society that thinks of expansion and monopoly of power as its central values. No matter how much we advise young people to take the time to find balance, it's not easy for those who are chasing after success. At that age, wanting to grow and expand is a physiological imperative. It does no good to talk to a tree in the fullness of its green youth about the beauty of autumn leaves dyed golden; it wouldn't want to abandon its green for the shades of autumn.

That's why harmony is needed. Young people should challenge themselves ambitiously and work with focus; we naturally need material security and success. Problems occur when material values are accepted as the only worthwhile ones. Human values are disappearing while we place absolute importance on success, expansion, and growth alone. Enlightened elders are the ones who can act as a counterweight in a society that is moving toward extremes.

In a success-centered society, only the roles of youth and young adulthood—like production, expansion, and development—are seen as important. When youth and middle age pass, these roles pass on to the next generation, and the cycle continues unabated. Many of the social problems we face now are intimately connected with this value system. In these times, relaxation and exhalation, giving and sharing are needed throughout society as well as in our personal lives. Retired people usually withdraw from productive activities, but instead of becoming bystanders or surplus humans, they can joyfully accept new roles—roles of instilling the value of completion, wisdom, tolerance, and caring in a society that places importance only on ceaseless expansion and development. When the younger generation is closing its fist and inhaling, the older generation needs to open its fist and exhale. Just as our hearts circulate blood through our bodies, going with the natural rhythm of contraction and relaxation, elders with enlightened consciousness should enable a balance between the two values of success and completion.

I see a balance of success and completion in the Way of New Life Forest at Earth Village in New Zealand. All kinds of trees live together in harmony in this forest. Massive black hoof mushrooms grow at the base of immense pine trees. Huge ferns with luxurious leaves grow in the shade of tall Kauri trees. And all kinds of mosses find a place in the shade of those ferns. Vines use the solid trunks of other trees as support, growing in symbiosis as if they were one body. The beauty of different organisms living in harmony, accepting and embracing each other, is deeply moving.

A New Future for Humanity

The older generation has the responsibility to show the younger generation that a valuable, beautiful old age is possible. We must demonstrate with our lives that there is more to life than the vigorous growth of people in their teens and 20s or the dynamic success drama of people in their 30s, 40s, and 50s. They need to see the beautiful drama of attaining internal maturity from the 60s onward. Seniors have a responsibility to show that the completion of their personal lives contributes to making a more humane and mature society, and they have the potential and power to do that.

Deciding to live to be 120 doesn't mean that you merely want to live a long time; it's an expression of your conviction and will to change your life, change your community, and set the human species and the earth on course to a better future. Therefore, I would like to see many people have such a dream and design their present and future through the choice to live to be 120 years old, just as I did. You might as well have a dream that can deeply move your soul, a dream so great that you have to live to 120 to realize it.

I believe in the power of the dreams that people have. Great, beautiful dreams make great, beautiful people. The great dream of one person could stop with changing his or her life, but a great dream embraced by many people could change the world. I see a tremendous human spirit in all the people I meet—great heroes and the extraordinary beings inside all ordinary individuals. Everyone has a desire for other people and life forms, as well as themselves, to be healthy and happy and to contribute to creating a better world. In particular, the older generation who are living out the second half of their lives—people like Sensei Hanabuchi—feel that all people are their own sons or daughters, and they have a deep sense of responsibility for humanity and the world. I think that we should consider those attitudes precious and ensure that they are revealed and reflected in our lives.

This is the first time in the history of the planet that the choices of each person will have such a decisive impact on the future of the earth. In previous generations, the power of individual choices was too insignificant to affect the whole planet. Now, thanks to the development of science and technology, we can sit in our living rooms and know what is happening on the other side of the planet. In most democratic countries, individuals are given the power to create political, social, and cultural change. Now we see what's happening around the globe, not just right around us, and we worry about our entire species and the whole planet, not just ourselves. This means that our consciousness is expanding—and this is, in fact, incredible progress in the history of our species. It's an awareness-expanding opportunity for each of us to transcend the limits of our individual thinking, to expand our consciousness infinitely.

The old age we will be experiencing has significance unprecedented in human history. We don't yet know how to live well for so long; role models for this situation are rare. We are attempting new things as we go back and forth between the ideas about aging we inherited from previous generations and the infinite potential unfolding before us.

American Baby Boomers who are now seniors have massive power—politically, economically, socially, and culturally—that cannot be compared with previous generations. The older generation not only has plenty of time but also the passion to pour their energy into meaningful work. If this power, time, and passion can be harnessed in the right direction, it will have an influence on individuals and, on a larger scale, the whole earth. We must believe in the power and wisdom of seniors to make that possible.

What today's seniors, the longest-lived generation in the history of our species, can leave on this earth will be determined by the values they pursue and how they live. A completely new perspective on old age could be established, depending on how each of us spends our later years, and a culture of wisdom never before seen in human history could be born. I hope that many people living in their old age, including me, will accept these historic roles and challenges and be able to create a new culture of aging. It is not government, industry, technology, or systems that can change society and save the earth. Each of us individually must choose to do so. That will soon create a new culture of aging, one that will act as a powerful force for changing the world.

If we pursue inner values and maturity of character and head toward completion in the latter half of our lives, and if we live lives of sharing and giving, we will be able to leave behind a healthier, happier, more peaceful, and more sustainable planet than the earth of today. Then we will be able to stand before the next generation with dignity, as true elders. With confidence and pride, we will be able to say, "We tried not to leave you with a polluted environment, we worked to create a kinder, gentler, and more humane world, and we hope that you will work to leave the generation that follows you with a better quality of life than we had."

" A completely new perspective
on old age could be
established, depending on
how each of us spends our later
years, and a culture of wisdom
never before seen in human
history could be born."

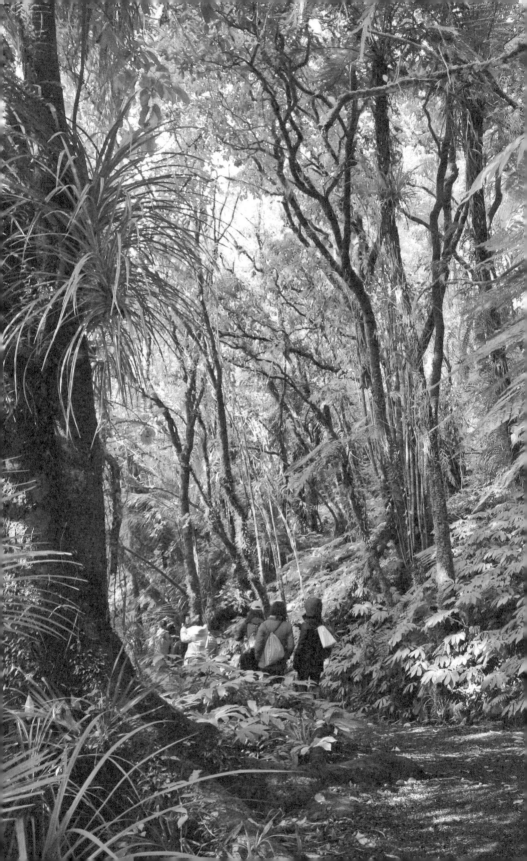

A Special Invitation to Earth Village

Writing this book has been a blessing to me. Like many people, I've experienced lots of difficulties in my life. But I've realized that the hardships, along with the joys, have made me who I am today. I've grown stronger and have come to love my life more as I've gone through all those moments. I now know my true identity more clearly and understand more fully the value and purpose of my life. This book has further increased my hope for humanity, because it is for people who, like you, want to live the second half of life according to their higher selves.

I want to make a suggestion. It involves something known as the gap year. This term commonly refers to the practice of taking a year off from studies between high school and college for various social experiences and self-development. Unfortunately, most formal education today is far removed from self-development. In fact, schools often steal selfhood from children. There is nothing so heart-rending as watching children give up hope for themselves and the world after losing confidence and self-respect through the process of endless competition.

In South Korea, I created the Benjamin School for Character Education to teach children life truths and skills that aren't taught in most schools. This one-year course is a kind of gap-year program for high school students. There are five things the school does not have: daily attendance, teachers, textbooks, tests, and homework. The number one rule is that you make a plan for what you will do and then act on that plan. Students set a project for themselves that they want to do and that will help other people and then complete it in one year. The self-respect, self-confidence, and self-worth they develop in this process will last their entire lives. It changes their destinies.

I think that people getting ready for or living in their period of completion (i.e., the second half of their lives) need a kind of gap year. It doesn't necessarily have to be one year in length. It could be several weeks or several months, or it could be even longer than a year. However long it is, I would like them to take that time to focus entirely on themselves, calmly looking back over the first half of their lives and then designing the second half.

And if you have the opportunity, I hope you will visit Earth Village in Kerikeri, New Zealand. There are two major projects underway at Earth Village. One is establishing a school where people from all over the world can stay for a few weeks or a few months, experiencing for themselves what it means to live as Earth Citizens and growing into Earth Citizen leaders themselves. Here they will learn natural health practices and life skills that let them be self-sufficient in health, happiness, and peace, and they will be reinvigorated as they train mind and body in nature. They will also experience raising vegetables and animals, building houses, and acquiring nature-friendly life skills. Participants will learn how to create and manage their lives as they want, using the creativity of their brains. I am picturing many Earth Citizen leaders training in this place and then returning to their communities to share what they have learned, changing their lives and communities in positive ways.

The second project being carried out at Earth Village is the New Zealand Meditation Tour. This is designed to allow participants to look back on their lives and to embrace the dream of Chunhwa as they design their lives going forward. The goal of the Meditation Tour is different from that of ordinary sightseeing, which is about viewing and enjoying natural beauty. This is a journey toward people's true selves, a journey for redesigning their lives.

Finding your true self is hard when your mind is chaotic and bound to reality. It's important to escape for a time from the treadmill and repeated patterns of your daily life. You're moving to a new time and space. Entering an entirely new environment gives your brain a jolt. In place of the habitual thought patterns it has always used, your brain starts to have new ideas and form new circuits. The very experience of flying from the Northern Hemisphere to New Zealand in the Southern Hemisphere will stimulate your brain. As you cross the earth's equator, you'll feel, "I really am living on the earth." You'll enter an unknown land, a new space and time. Virtually unblemished nature, as you encounter it in New Zealand, will fill and renew your body, mind, and consciousness—your everything.

Earth Village in New Zealand has an extraordinary energy. The crisp, exhilarating air is like none you've breathed anywhere else on earth. The adjectives clear and clean come nowhere close to describing it; somehow it fills and revitalizes your whole body. In the woods of Earth Village, all you have to do is sit there and breath. You wonder how your breathing can be so deep and why you just want to keep taking those fresh, deep breaths. Every time you inhale, you feel refreshing air coming deep into your lungs, into every nook and cranny of your brain, and you get the feeling that it's cleaning and healing all the cells of your body. I call this the clean lung effect and the clean brain effect.

A botanist who came to the woodland path at Earth Village said that this place hosts the 10 species of plants that give off the most phytoncides, natural antibiotics they emit to protect themselves from pests and pathogenic bacteria. For humans, phytoncides are natural healing substances that relieve stress, strengthen heart and lung function, and have a germicidal effect.

Although the natural environment of Earth Village is special, what makes it different from the natural setting anywhere else in New Zealand is the presence of spirit. It is the spirit of Chunhwa, the spirit of Earth Citizens. Earth Village is truly a place for learning and experiencing Chunhwa, a place that lets us feel an earnest desire for Chunhwa. As I thought of the many people who would visit this place from around the world, I developed sites for Chunhwa meditation in various locations, and I gave them names containing the meaning of Chunhwa.

One of these places is Chunhwa Park. Three waterfalls there represent heaven, earth, and humanity. In this book, I have included photographs of the beautiful scenery at those waterfalls, but they cannot adequately convey the real, vibrant energy of the place. In a primal forest that preserves pristine nature in its divine splendor, all the cells in your body are filled by the sounds of the waterfalls, the streams rushing through ravines, and the birds as well as by the life energy of nature that pours out of the mossy rocks, the ground, and the trees. If you close your eyes and meditate there for a while, you will automatically feel that heaven, earth, and humanity have entered into you, and you are all one through energy.

While soaking in this splendor, you can contemplate how far you have come and where you are going as you climb each of the 120 steps of the Completion of the Soul, a stairway surrounded by primeval forest. When you sit on a broad wooden deck at the end of the path, you will be able to feel divine energy pouring down into the crown of your head like a waterfall, and you will be inspired to choose a 120-year life.

Not far from Earth Village, you will encounter a majestic, 1,000-year-old hwangchil tree (*Dendropanax*), which has an overwhelming life force. That tree may give you this message: "Welcome to this place. I've been waiting for you. May you achieve the dream of Chunhwa and make a better world."

I tell people who come on a Meditation Tour to bring with them an earnest *hwadu*, a question to solve. If you have a problem you want to resolve, a problem that you haven't been able to clear up no matter how hard you've thought about it, that is a hwadu. You will receive a clear message, one that matches the earnestness of your desire for an answer to the questions you've been struggling with.

That happens on its own when you're one with nature, not by thinking about it. The layers of defenses surrounding you will fall away when the life energy of nature, entering your body through deep breathing, opens up all your energy points. Your jumbled thoughts will stop, and you will be able to watch yourself honestly as the energy of your emotions is purified. Your consciousness will automatically be uplifted when the unsullied energy of nature fills the spot left empty by your emotions and thoughts.

When the nature inside and outside of you become one, you will hear the messages you need, and the wholeness that has always been in you will awaken. Finding and developing that wholeness or completeness is the process of Chunhwa, completion of the soul. You will truly be able to start a life of Chunhwa when you have encountered a whole new self beyond what you had been thinking of as "me." You will discover the true self that had always been hidden deep within you, beyond your thoughts and emotions. That is your true value, the value of humanity, the value of life.

The New Zealand Meditation Tour is a time for the ego to face itself, a time for the caterpillar to transform within its cocoon. If a chick is to emerge from its egg, it must bravely peck away at the shell. In the same way, we must unhesitatingly choose to design new lives for ourselves. We may have been living as our environments demanded, according to social systems. Although we have lived our lives diligently so far, we all want to design new lives for ourselves if given the opportunity. Everyone has a desire to live a life based on higher values, to transcend their previous thoughts, memories, and habits. Hope revives inside us when we encounter that beautiful, perfect, true self. And when hope for ourselves revives, it can become hope for the world.

As I've been developing Earth Village, I've come to have confidence that this place will really be a land that creates a new zeal. When you come to Earth Village, a pure longing to live your life loving others wells up naturally in your heart. You feel a passion for saving yourself and for becoming the hope of the earth and all humanity. That longing is the greatest gift you can give your brain. When we have that dream, our brains find a reason and purpose for living to be 120 years old. Our brains start designing a life of Chunhwa, the life of completion we really want. I want to enable everyone who visits Earth Village to find that dream and that passion. That is why I am creating Earth Village and why I want to spend the rest of my life working for something to leave behind for the world, for people, for the earth.

All of our lives are beautiful and brilliant right now, at this very moment. They will shine even more brightly if we feel and wholeheartedly choose what we will use our life energy for until we die. I offer you my deepest respect and gratitude for all the good deeds you have done so far for yourself and others. All the things we have done have come together to make this world a better place, and I believe our actions will do that in the future, too. Our life energy inevitably runs out with time. How will we use our remaining energy? That is what's important. We might as well use that life energy to passionately achieve our dreams. What do you think? I'm sincerely and excitedly looking forward to what we will be able to leave behind in this world as we use our precious life energy, brilliantly and beautifully, in the time we have left.

I would like to thank you for reading this book, and I hope that my thinking about a life of completion will help you lead a richer life. May your life be full of the joy of completion, a 120-year life of aging beautifully as you achieve your dreams in good health and happiness.

From Earth Village in New Zealand,
Ilchi Lee

ACKNOWLEDGMENTS

Many people helped in the creation of this book or gave it their support. To them all, I am truly grateful.

Hyerin Moon and Jiyoung Oh at Best Life Media put their editing and production expertise into it from beginning to end. Daniel Graham translated it into English, and Nicole Dean and Phyllis Elving transformed the English into engaging text that's easy to read. Sue Vander Hook gave the manuscript its final proofreading polish. Dr. Deborah Coady provided valuable feedback that guided the editing process, and Michela Mangiaracina helped with the final stages of book production. Hyerin Moon and Jordan Diamond contributed the beautiful photos of New Zealand that you find throughout the book, and Jooyoung Ryu contributed the warm illustrations.

A number of people who are in the second half of their lives shared their stories and ideas on successful aging: Susan Gerace, Alyse Gutter, Anne Covert, Sandra Scheer, David Plummer, Janet Duda, Brian O'Reilly, Marti Bay, Joy Venegas, and Susan Propst. Although I could not include all of them in the book, their lives and dedication to their communities inspired me and shine as examples for others.

And to all of the enlightened elders who gave their endorsement to this book—Barbara Marx Hubbard, don Miguel Ruiz, Neale Donald Walsch, Michael Bernard Beckwith, Dr. Christiane Northrup, Dr. Emeran Mayer, Dr. Reed Tuckson, Dr. Jessie Jones, Dr. Darrell Wolfe—I am humbled by your words and am sincerely grateful.

ABOUT THE AUTHOR

Ilchi Lee is an impassioned visionary, educator, mentor, and innovator; he has dedicated his life to teaching energy principles and researching and developing methods to nurture the full potential of the human brain.

For more than 35 years, his life's mission has been to help people harness their own creative power and personal potential. For this goal, he has developed many successful mind-body training methods, including Body & Brain Yoga and Brain Education. His principles and methods have inspired many people around the world to live healthier and happier lives.

Lee is a *New York Times* bestselling author who has penned more than 40 books, including *The Call of Sedona: Journey of the Heart*, *Change: Realizing Your Greatest Potential*, and *The Power Brain: Five Steps to Upgrading Your Brain Operating System*.

He is also a well-respected humanitarian who has been working with the United Nations and other organizations for global peace. He began the Earth Citizen Movement, a global drive to raise awareness of the values of earth citizenship and put them into practice.

Lee serves as president of the University of Brain Education, the Global Cyber University, and the International Brain Education Association. For more information about Ilchi Lee and his work, visit ilchi.com.

RESOURCES

Body & Brain Yoga and Tai Chi Classes

The 100 Body & Brain Yoga and Tai Chi centers in the United States are one of the best ways you can make the exercises and principles introduced in this book a meaningful part of your daily life. They offer classes, workshops, and individual sessions based on East Asian healing and energy philosophies. The expert instructors and center community also provide advice and support for your continued growth and life creation.

Special Offer for the Readers of This Book

Bring a copy of *I've Decided to Live 120 Years* to a Body & Brain Yoga and Tai Chi center anywhere in the United States and get 50% off an Introductory Session. During this 45-minute private session, an instructor will check your flexibility, balance, breathing, energy, and stress levels and recommend a customized practice plan tailored to your physical, mental, emotional, and/or spiritual needs.

This special offer ends December 31, 2019.

Find a center near you at BodynBrain.com.

Retreats and Workshops

Opportunities to immerse yourself in the feeling of being one with nature, reflect on your life, and plan for its second half are offered at these retreat centers.

Sedona Mago Retreat

Nestled among the red rocks on a stunning, 175-acre stretch of land under the wide blue sky of the high Arizonan desert, Sedona Mago Retreat is an ideal place for letting nature sweep aside the hustle and bustle of a busy life. Here you will have a chance to look within to find the answers to who you are and what you really want. Go for a personal retreat to plan the second half of your life or join one of the many programs for ongoing self-development offered there. Learn more at **SedonaMagoRetreat.org**.

Honor's Haven

For a personal getaway among the rolling hills of the Shawangunk Mountain Region, the gateway to the Catskills in New York, visit Honor's Haven Resort & Spa. The 200 acres of lush gardens, crystalline lake, and meditative forest will inspire you to discover the greater you within. Enjoy wellness classes and retreat programs in which experienced instructors will guide you on your inner journey. Learn more at **HonorsHaven.com**.

Online Resources

Live 120 Years Special Online Course

I've Decided to Live 120 Years springs to life in this online course. Its meditation and writing exercises walk you through the key ideas and practices featured in the book. It includes exclusive interviews with Ilchi Lee and other experts. Readers receive a special discount for the course. For more information, visit **Live120YearsCourse.com**.

Free Resources at Live120YearsBook.com

Author Ilchi Lee developed a handful of free resources to help readers incorporate what they learned from this book into their daily lives. Visit **Live120YearsBook.com** to access these free resources. They include the following and more:

For Your Physical Power
- Illustrated, step-by-step Longevity Walking guide
- Body & Brain Yoga stretching exercise video

For Your Heart Power
- Energy sensitizing exercise video
- Guided nature meditation audio files

For Your Brain Power
- 5 Ways to Improve Your Brain Power guide
- Brain Wave Vibration exercise video

One-Minute Exercise App

Author Ilchi Lee had an app developed to help you adopt One-Minute Exercise as a daily habit. Available for both iOS and Android, it includes an alarm, timer, tracker, and library of One-Minute Exercise videos to follow. You can learn more about the One Minute Change app and download it for free at **1MinuteChange.com**.

Earth Citizen Movement

Living as an Earth Citizen begins with each individual's choice, but when many individuals come together, systemic change can begin. The Earth Citizen Movement raises awareness of the power of personal choice, promotes the spirit of earth citizenship, and spearheads real action for a healthier and sustainable world. It is coordinated by the Earth Citizens Organization (ECO), a nonprofit that trains Earth Citizen leaders and introduces ways to live mindfully and sustainably. You can learn more about an Earth Citizen lifestyle, find volunteer opportunities, join an Earth Citizen Club, and see ECO training programs at **EarthCitizens.org**.